XH-1 Therapy

by

Dr. Laiyin Yan

DORRANCE PUBLISHING CO., INC.
PITTSBURGH, PENNSYLVANIA 15222

ISBN # 0-8059-4088-X
Printed in the United States of America

First Printing

For information or to order additional books, please write:
Dorrance Publishing Co., Inc.
643 Smithfield Street
Pittsburgh, Pennsylvania 15222
U.S.A.

Contents

Foreword

January 17, 1994

XH-1 therapy was originally applied for treating twenty-one types of illnesses such as headache, migraine, dizziness, glaucoma, chest pain, tight chest, palpitation, pain and swelling of joints, back pain, sprain, and cervical disorders. For rescuing critically ill patients, including those with acute heart failure and acute renal failure, it can quickly relieve each of the patients' ailments at no less than a 90 percent efficacy rate. For treating chronic renal failure, it can have some of the patients under fifty years of age, after one to two months of treatment, no longer needing a kidney transplant or kidney dialysis. And, after six months to one year of treatment, their health has been basically rehabilitated.

Since 1987, Bangkok Metropolitan Administration applied the XH-1 therapy for not just treating illnesses but also for treating drug addiction and solved the world's most difficult-to-solve problems of treating drug addiction. A total of at least fifty thousand illness and drug addiction cases were treated at efficacy rates of no less than 90 percent on both treating illnesses and treating drug addiction. It also successfully rescued 117 patients with severe heroin withdrawal reaction and eliminated mortality cases due to the severe-withdrawal-reaction-caused acute heart failure and rupture-and-hemorrhage of capillaries of the spasmatic internal organs. During the use of this therapy, there has never been any negative medical incident nor any adverse effect. This therapy is deeply welcomed by the truly motivated drug quitters. Now the XH-1 therapy is already being used in every medical and narcotic clinic of Bangkok Metropolitan Administration.

This book introduces the principles and applications of XH-1 therapy and also heavily introduces the Bangkok Metropolitan Administration's four whole years, from 1987 to 1990, of experimental reports on XH-1 illness and drug-addiction treatment, with the main point focused on observing and analyzing 100-case heroin quitters, and proves that XH-1 therapy's therapeutic effect on treating illnesses and drug addiction includes the following:

1. In fifteen minutes, it can relieve heroin quitters' seventeen withdrawal symptoms.
2. It can effectively suppress heroin quitters' usual climax of the severe withdrawal reacted on the third and fourth days.
3. It can quickly return heroin users' six worst items of health condition to health baseline level after seven days of health-recovery treatment.

XH-1 therapy achieved at least 90 percent efficacy rate on solving the above three most vital key problems of treating heroin-drug addiction.

The process of the clinical experiment and the writing of this textbook was assisted by the Bangkok Metropolitan Administration of Thailand, U.S. Department of Health and Human Services; California Medical Research Institute of U.S.A.; Department of Health and Ministry of Foreign Affairs of the Republic of China; and some countries' related embassies or representative offices of the Republic of China; ministries of health of the following countries: Kingdom of Tonga, Nauru, Tuvalu, Vietnam, etc.; and the related government leaders and medical experts: Deputy Permanent Secretary on Public Health of Bangkok Metropolitan Administration-Dr. Kachit Choopanya; person in charge of the twelfth Narcotic Clinic of Bangkok Metropolitan Administration Ms. Suneeporn Anuttarakulvanich; Director of Office of Program Coordination and Review and Office for Substance Abuse Prevention, U.S. Department of Health and Human Services Dr. Yuth Nimit; Royal physician of Kingdom of Tonga and advisor of California Medical Research Institute of U.S.A. Dr. Tili Puloka; and Mr. Peter Shieh of California Medical Research Institute of U.S.A. Many thanks to them.

Dr. Laiyin Yan
Research Professor and Vice-President of
California Medical Research Institute, U.S.A.
Advisor for the Drug Addicts Treatment Program
Bangkok Metropolitan Administration, Thailand

Permanent Address:
64/65 Tiwanon Rd., Nonthaburi, 11000 Thailand

June 14, 1996

Dr. Laiyin Yan
1536 Stevens Ave.
San Gabriel
CA 91776, U.S.A.

Dear Dr. Yan,

Congratulations on your receipt of the U.S. Government's
approval with the position of world's most outstanding and
famous doctor and the most honorable Ell qualification to
immigrate into the United States.

I also want to congratulate you on the completion of your
book "XH-1 Therapy". I believe its publication will allow
even more people understand and benefit from it.

Hopefully you will continue to assist the Government of
Thailand to use the XH-1 therapy to treat ailments and drug
addiction.

Sincerely yours,

Dr. Kachit Choopanya
M.D.,M.P.H.,M.P.H. & T.M. (Tulane) U.S.A.
Deputy Governor of Bangkok Metropolitan Administration

March 7, 1996

Dr. Laiyin Yan
1536 Stevens Ave.
San Gabriel
CA 91776, U.S.A.

Dear Dr. Yan,

When I was the person in charge of the Drug Addicts Treatment
Center and the vice-president of Department of Health in
Bangkok Metropolitan Administration, I have used the XH-1
therapy to treat ailments and drug addiction and obtained
very good results.

In Geneva's international drug addicts treatment conference,
I have introduced the XH-1 therapy and have received attention
given from all.

I am congratulating on the book you wrote, "XH-1 Therapy"
for being published soon. It provides the work of drug
addicts treatment a new and effective method of treatment.

Sincerely yours,

Dr. Suphak Vanichseni

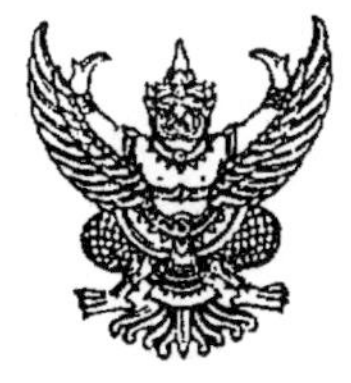

Drug Abuse Prevention and
Treatment Div., Health Dept.,
BMA.

March 7, 1996

Dr. Laiyin Yan

1536 Stevens Ave.
San Gabriel
CA 91776, USA.

Dear Dr. Yan

    First of all let me congratulate on your new position as a President of California Medical Research Institute, and a completion of book-writing "XH-1 therapy". It is really a good news and a great pleasure.

    I do believe on both what you have contributed to our drug addicts and the "XH-1 therapy" which will be mostly beneficial to our drug prevention and treatment services of the Bangkok Metropolitan Administration as a whole.

    May I take this opportunity to convey our thankfulness for your cooperation and do certainly expect to receive this remarkable success from you whether in terms of educational research or the opportunity for study tour & training in your institution.

    We will be most happy if any time you might have come to visit us and you are always welcome to our organization.

    Once again thank you and congratulation,

    Kind regards.

Yours sincerely,

Dr. Suwanee Raktham
Director

Introducing the XH-1 Illness and Drug-Addiction Therapy

According to centuries-old Chinese medical qigong therapeutic theory, using specified signals to work on related locations on the skin surfaces will allow the qi and blood to flow freely, and the body's mechanism and the functions of the related locations will rehabilitate to normal and by relieving illnesses and pains to achieve the purpose of treating illnesses and drug addiction. According to Bangkok Metropolitan Administration documents, for four years, the therapy treated illnesses and drug addiction on over fifty-thousand people, had no adverse effects, and the efficacy rate reached over 90 percent.

The Medication-Free XH-1 Illness and Drug-Addiction Therapy.

The Main and Present Method of Treating Drug-Addiction in Narcotic Clinics of Thailand.

In the meantime, the methods of treating drug addiction in Thailand's narcotic clinics mainly included the medication therapy provided by the United Nations. The therapy takes thirty days, and the medication dosage reduces according to the progress. The medication itself, such as Methadone, however, is a harmful substance to human beings. It can be easy to become addicted and hard to quit. Therefore the drug quitters have to come continuously to the drug rehabilitation clinic every day to take the medication. If they stop taking the medication, they will suffer from withdrawal symptoms similar to the withdrawal symptoms of drugs, although less severe and with no life-threatening danger.

Drug Addicts' Illnesses and Pains.

Besides the influences from the society, one reason a big portion of people take drugs is because they have illnesses, such as stomach pain, headaches, or pain of the limb joints. After being referred by others, these people started taking heroin and other narcotic drugs to stop the pain and ended up addicted to drugs.

Due to the chronic usage of drugs, the health of a large portion of the drug addicts were harmed and, therefore, ended up having several illnesses.

To Treat Drug Addiction One Must First Relieve Illnesses and Pains.

The present drug addiction treating method, which uses medication, ignores the treatment for the addicts' illnesses and pains, whether they are drug induced or non-drug induced. Because some of the drug quitters are continuously having illnesses and pains, they have to use drugs continuously in order to relieve them.

Entering the Golden Triangle to Probe Drug Addicts' Phenomenon of Illnesses and Pains.

In order to research extensively the drug addicts' symptoms, special signs, and patterns of pain and illnesses and figure out how to find an effective way to treat illnesses and drug addiction, I risked my life and entered the Golden Triangle of Burma in 1985 all by myself for over one year to investigate and research. After the investigation and research, I have known that drug addicts possess the following illnesses.

1. There are seventeen withdrawal symptoms: 1) headache, 2) dizziness, 3) drowsiness, 4) yawning, 5) sneezing, 6) neck pain, 7) back and spinal pain, 8) lumbar pain, 9) muscle cramp of limbs, 10) abdominal pain, 11) cramp of internal organs, 12) nausea, 13) tight chest, 14) chest pain, 15) palpitation, 16) cold sweat with cold hands and feet, and 17) weakness.
2. When the patient is having a severe reaction of withdrawal symptoms, and the suffering is not controlled immediately, he will very quickly suffer from spasm and hemorrhage of the internal organs and cardiac failure and, thus, die.
3. Drug addicts suffer from many more illnesses than normal people.

After research and investigation, if one is going to treat drug use effectively, he must first relieve the drug addicts' illnesses and pains, whether they are drug induced or non-drug induced.

Probing the Possibilities of Using Chinese Herbs to Treat Illnesses and Drug Addiction.

I have tried using the Chinese herbs to treat drug addiction and discovered that:

1. Drug addicts suffered from more illnesses, in both severity and variety, than normal people.
2. During the third to fourth day of withdrawal, the drug quitters will suffer from severe withdrawal symptoms, accompanied by life-threatening danger. It is very difficult to eliminate the danger by Chinese herbs in a short period of time.
3. By using Chinese herbs to treat illnesses and drug addiction, the patient has to be hospitalized so that when there are severe withdrawal symptoms, the condition can be observed and handled by appropriate procedures to avoid the life-threatening danger. Hospitalization itself, however, is expensive.
4. It takes a group of experienced Chinese-herbal physicians to execute the work of drug-addiction treatment.

Because of the above circumstances, massively executing and promoting the use of Chinese herbs to treat drug addiction is very difficult.

Probing the Possibility of Using Acupuncture to Treat Illnesses and Drug Addiction.

According to the principles of using acupuncture to relieve illnesses, at the Golden Triangle I have used acupuncture to treat illnesses and drug addiction and have obtained good results. This has increased my confidence in treating illnesses and drug addiction. However, during the third and fourth days of withdrawal, most of the drug quitters' withdrawal symptoms have a very severe reaction and are life-threatening; it is hard to apply only acupuncture as a means of emergency life rescue. And when the withdrawal symptoms are very severe, the patient's whole body suffers from spasms, twisting and rolling around; therefore, it is hard to apply needles.

Probing the Possibilities of Using the Electrical Acupuncture Instrument and Qigong-Signal Therapeutic Instrument to Treat Illnesses and Drug Addiction.

For quitting smoking and alcoholism, using the electrical acupuncture instrument or qigong-signal instrument is, indeed, a very successful method. However, when the withdrawal symptoms become severe, the patients can have spasms all over the body, hemorrhage of internal organs, and heart failure and, consequently, die. Most of the electrical acupuncture instruments available from the market are dangerous to the heart and blood pressure; therefore I do not dare to use it. Most of the qigong-signal instruments require that, during the treatment, patients must relax and concentrate their mind on their Dantien (the upper two-thirds of the line joining the umbilicus and symphysis pubis). However, when the withdrawal symptoms become severe, the patients' bodies suffer from spasms. When twisting and rolling around, they are not able to relax and work with this therapy. And most of the electrical acupuncture instruments and qigong-signal instruments are not equipped with features to perform emergency life rescue.

Developing a Kind of New Medication-Free XH-1 Illness and Drug-Addiction Therapy.

After observations and research, I have finally developed a kind of therapy, which is done by placing electrodes of the XH-1 rehabilitation therapeutic machine (invented by myself) on the related locations of the skin. This therapy achieves the effect of treating illnesses and drug addiction without the use of medication.

This illness and drug-addiction therapy is able to eliminate the severe withdrawal symptoms before they happen and not let them happen at all. It is also able to rescue the patients with the severe withdrawal symptoms that are already happening. In most cases, after five to fifteen minutes of therapy, the danger of the withdrawal symptoms is relieved. This illness and drug-addiction therapy has no danger to the human body.

Our therapy for treating illnesses and drug addiction includes two main contents:

1. The XH-1 rehabilitation therapeutic machine I invented myself.
2. A medication-free illness and drug-addiction therapy developed according to the study of qigong.

Our main point for this illness and drug-addiction therapy goes as follows. First, it mainly relieves the drug addicts' illnesses, whether they are drug induced or non-drug induced; therefore it is able to reach the goal of treating illnesses and drug addiction and then is followed by further treatment to rehabilitate the drug quitters' health so that they can live and work like normal people.

The principles of this illness and drug-addiction therapy are to use a special signal on certain locations on the skin to restore the functions all over the body back to normal, such as the heart, blood pressure, nervous system, etc., to eliminate the seventeen illnesses associated with the withdrawal symptoms described before. Therefore this therapy prevents mortality caused by the spasm and hemorrhage of internal organs and heart failure and also, at the same time, relieves other illnesses and pains, whether they are drug induced or non-drug induced, in order to reach the goal of treating illnesses and drug addiction.

Results of Using the XH-1 Illness and Drug-Addiction Therapy.

For four years since January 1, 1987, in Thailand, this medication-free XH-1 illness and drug-addiction therapy has treated over fifty thousand patients, including those who are not drug addicts. According to the statistics from the Department of Health, Bangkok Metropolitan Administration, the efficacy of this therapy has reached over 90 percent. All the clinical statistic data are stored into the computer file of Bangkok Metropolitan Administration.

Special Features of the XH-1 Illness and Drug-Addiction Therapy.

Four years of clinical usage proved that XH-1 illness and drug addiction therapy has the following special features.

1. Within a short period of five to fifteen minutes, it is able to relieve the drug quitters' illnesses and pains and relieve the severe life-threatening symptoms of withdrawal and therefore effectively rescue many drug quitters' lives. There has been no mortality during the treatment of drug addiction for all four years.
2. Within four to seven days, it is able to completely relieve the seventeen illnesses of withdrawal symptoms and relieve the suffering of the drug quitters due to illnesses, whether these illnesses are drug induced or non-drug induced.
3. After the treatment for drug addiction, followed by seven more days of health-recovery treatment, most drug quitters are having a good food appetite, good sleep, good spirit after awakening, good physical strength, strengthened sexual function, and a comfortable feel and are able to live and work like normal people.
4. This therapy has a speedy effectiveness on adjusting the body functions, driving them toward normal, and, therefore, relieving the symptoms. Besides using this therapy for treating drug addiction, it can also be used for emergency rescue, treating illnesses, and rehabilitating health.
5. The biggest feature of this therapy is that the more obvious the symptoms or pains are, the more conspicuous the effectiveness of this

therapy is.

6. This therapy treats illnesses, drug addiction, and life-threatening emergencies without using medication. Therefore it can save a large amount of medication and cost.
7. The use of this therapy is simple. Therefore, in our clinic, the new drug quitters or regular patients need only one instruction to know how to use it, so they can apply this therapy on themselves when they come for the next visits.
8. This therapy has no danger. When patients apply the therapy on themselves, sometimes they do not place the electrodes at the exact right places. At most, this will reduce the effectiveness of the therapy, but it has no danger.

Principles of the XH-1 Illness and Drug-Addiction Therapy.

The Miraculous Qigong.

From the hospitals, television, or qigong performing meetings, we see some qigong masters point their hands to send qi energy at the patients' ill or painful parts of their bodies, and the patients' pains or illnesses are relieved or eliminated! This is too miraculous! What exactly is qi itself?

The Essence of Qi.

In 1978 the Shanghai Chinese Medical Research Institute and Gu Hangsheng of Shanghai Nuclear Physics Research Institute cooperated. They detected what the external qi, sent from the qigong masters, really is. It is a kind of infrared electromagnetic wave with a fluctuation of 85 percent. From then on, it is proven that qi is a kind of electromagnetic wave. The traveling of the electrons is the fundamental substance of qi.

Differences between the External Qi Sent from Qigong Masters.

In 1979 Yan Laiyin (Xiao Huiheng) of Shanghai Chinese Medical Research Institute specifically detected the wave characteristics of the external qi sent by qigong masters and found out that the wave forms and sections of the external qi sent from each of the qigong masters are different from each other. The wave form of the external qi sent from each qigong master also differs according to his health and the environmental conditions. They also have found out that what some of the qigong masters sent out are magnetic fields or static fields. When applying these qi to humans, they had different reactions clinically. Some qi can treat illnesses with good results, but some other qi can cause chills, sweating, wheezing, tight chest, palpitation, and other adverse effects. Their similarity is, however, that all the external qi sent have fluctuating electromagnetic waves.

The World's First Qigong-Signal Therapeutic Instrument, Which Imitates the External Qi of Qigong, Was Awarded with an International Gold Medal.

The qigong masters who are able to treat certain illnesses with good results can only treat a few patients within a period of time. If the external qi of these qigong masters are imitated and programmed into a qigong-signal instrument to replace the qigong masters in treatment patients, then having thousands of qigong-signal instruments would be equivalent to having thousands of qigong masters treating the patients, thus solving the problems of the hard-to-get-hold-of (and in short-supply) qigong masters.

In 1981 Yan Laiyin (Xiao Huiheng) of Shanghai Chinese Medical Research Institute analyzed the wave form from a lot of external qi and have found out the wave forms that are able to treat certain illnesses conspicuously. They made the world's first magnetic-tape converting type of qigong-signal therapeutic instrument, which was approved at the end of 1981. The first ten instruments were sent to Beijin for the leaders of China, such as Yeh Jienyin and other leaders, to use. On March 22, 1982, the China Department of Health approved its mass production. In the meantime, it is estimated that there are hundreds of thousands of the qigong-signal therapeutic instruments being used in China with no adverse effect ever found. On January 15, 1989, this qigong-signal therapeutic instrument was awarded with Gold Medal from the International Traditional Rehabilitation Medical Conference. This instrument achieved an 85 percent efficacy rate on treating certain illnesses.

Characteristics and Essence of Qi.

There is a famous saying from Chinese medicine, "If qi and blood don't free flow, then pain appears." This is saying that the qi and blood inside the normal healthy person travel continuously, and if qi and blood free flow, then the person must be healthy. If qi and blood do not flow freely, then illness/pain appears. In the term *qi and blood*, the word *blood* obviously is the blood and the word *qi* stands for the traveling electrons inside the human body. The electrons of the normal human body travel at set patterns. The traveling of the electrons creates an electromagnetic wave. Therefore electromagnetic waves can be detected at various parts of the body, such as in the encephalogram, cardiogram, electrogastrogram, electromyogram, etc. If the person dies, then the electrons stop traveling, and the electronic wave on every part of the body disappears.

When the value of the electrical resistance and capacity of certain parts of the human body has an abnormal change, which means it is creating the qi and blood not flowing freely, the electronic wave would deviate from normal, and clinically this would show various type of illnesses.

The Principles of Applying the Internal Qi of Qigong to Treat Illnesses.

People who have mastered the qigong exercise all have a feeling in common. That is the sign of qi movement inside their bodies. According to modern scientific observation and research, it has proved that the movement of qi is the sign of electrons traveling inside the body. This type of qi, when it travels in various parts of the body, creates various types of electromagnetic waves. The wave forms of the internal qi between qigong masters are different. And the wave form of the internal qi of each qigong master himself differs under different health conditions or environments.

If qi and blood don't free flow, then pain appears, which also means various types of illnesses and pains appear. Blood is the "mother" of qi, and qi is the "leader" of blood, which means blood nourishes the qi, and qi moves the blood. Blood is the vice and qi the main. Therefore, throughout history people who have mastered qigong use their mind power to move the qi, which is the electron flow, to where the illnesses or pains are located, to free flow the qi and blood, to drive the abnormal electromagnetic wave to normal, and to achieve the goal of rehabilitating to normal mechanism of the body.

The Newest Invention, XH-1 Rehabilitation Therapeutic Machine, Which Imitates the Internal Qi of Qigong.

People who have mastered qigong can drive their own internal qi to achieve the goal of treating their own illnesses. This type of qi is the electrons traveling in the body and is a kind of electromagnetic wave. And the internal qi of everyone who mastered qigong has a different electromagnetic wave form. After analyzing a lot of the electromagnetic wave forms from the people who have mastered qigong, I have found a certain wave section that is effective in treating illnesses. By following this section of the wave, I made another type of new internal-qi imitating model, the XH-1 rehabilitation therapeutic machine.

XH-1 Rehabilitation Therapeutic Machine Has the Characteristics of Qigong Treatment.

According to the Chinese medical qigong therapeutic principles thousands of years ago, the new internal-qi imitating XH-1 rehabilitation therapeutic machine applies a specified signal on the related locations on the skin surface to make the qi and blood flow freely so the related parts of the body can be rehabilitated to normal and achieves the goal of treating illnesses and drug addiction by relieving illnesses and pains. This machine was clinically applied for more than four years at the Twelfth Narcotic Clinic of Bangkok Metropolitan Department of Health. They have found out that if using the therapeutic method of acupuncture to apply this therapeutic machine, it will not be able to rescue the life-threatening signs of the severe heroin withdrawal on time.

If using the therapeutic method of qigong to clinically apply this therapeutic machine to rescue the patients in life-threatening situations of severe heroine withdrawal reactions, it would only take five to fifteen minutes to save the patients from life-threatening danger and to be able to calm them down.

The Safety of Using the XH-1 Rehabilitation Therapeutic Machine to Treat Illnesses and Drug Addiction.

The average energy consumption of the XH-1 rehabilitation therapeutic machine is <1.6 milliwatt. Because it is working at extremely low consumption, its electrical parameter is very safe for the human body. The wave form, which the XH-1 rehabilitation therapeutic machine imitates, of the internal qi of people who have mastered qigong is one of the normal physiological parameters of the human body. For four years, the Bangkok Metropolitan Department of Health has used the XH-1 rehabilitation therapeutic machine to treat illnesses and drug addiction on over fifty thousand people, successfully rescued 117 patients who suffered from the severe withdrawal reaction, eliminated mortality, and never had any medical incident. According to the statistics from the Bangkok Metropolitan Department of Health, the efficacy rate of treating illnesses and drug addiction is over 90 percent.

XH-1 Rehabilitation Therapeutic Machine Has Conspicuous Therapeutic Effect on Twenty-one Types of Illnesses.

Besides being able to treat addiction to heroin, cocaine, amphetamines, and other drugs, the XH-1 rehabilitation therapeutic machine can also treat the following twenty-one illnesses with conspicuous effects: 1. certain heart diseases, 2. high blood pressure, 3. low blood pressure, 4. headache, 5. migraine, 6. dizziness, 7. Menier's Syndrome, 8. glaucoma, 9. insomnia, 10. neck pain, 11. stiff neck, 12. allergic rhinitis, 13. sprain, 14. back pain and soreness, 15. joint pain, 16. arthredema, 17. stomach disorders, 18. dysmenorrhea, 19. shoulder periarthritis, 20. child neo-myopia, and 21. strange diseases of which the etiology is unknown.

As far as deformity or infectious diseases are concerned, this therapy can only be considered as adjunctive.

There Are Three Designated Goals That Need to be Solved When Using XH-1 to Treat Heroin Addiction.

1. When heroin quitters' withdrawal reacts, whether the seventeen heroin withdrawal symptoms produced can be relieved immediately.
2. Whether heroin quitters' usual climax of the severe withdrawal reaction of the third and fourth days can be effectively suppressed.
3. Whether the heroin users' six worst items of health condition can be rehabilitated to a healthy level.

These are the three main designated goals of heroin-addiction treatment. Regardless of any kind of drug-addiction treatment, only if these three problems can be solved will the drug-addiction treatment be counted as successful.

The Clinical Technic Demand of Heroin-Addiction Treatment.

Observing the Conditions of Relieving Heroin Quitters' Seventeen Withdrawal Symptoms by the XH-1 Illnesses and Drug-Addiction Therapy.

Heroin quitters' seventeen withdrawal symptoms: 1) headache, 2) dizziness, 3) drowsiness, 4) yawning, 5) sneezing, 6) neck pain, 7) back and spinal pain, 8) lumbar pain, 9) muscle cramp of limbs, 10) abdominal pain, 11) cramp of internal organs, 12) nausea, 13) tight chest, 14) chest pain, 15) palpitation, 16) cold sweat with cold hands and feet, and 17) weakness.

Observing each subject's daily conditions of drug-addiction treatment.

Observing the group's total daily conditions of drug-addiction treatment.

Observing, during the seven-day course of drug-addiction treatment, XH-1'S therapeutic effect on each of the seventeen withdrawal symptoms.

Observing Whether XH-1 Illness and Drug-Addiction Therapy Can Effectively Suppress the Heroin Quitter's Usual Climax of the Severe Withdrawal Reaction of the Third and Fourth Days.

Observing whether the daily average number of types of each subject's withdrawal symptoms has a tendency to increase or decrease to assure whether XH-1 illness and drug-addiction therapy can effectively suppress the heroin quitter's usual climax of the severe withdrawal reactions of the third and fourth days.

Observing, during the course of drug-addiction treatment, whether the changing tendency of the three types of severity of heroin quitters' withdrawal symptoms has a tendency to increase or decrease to assure whether XH-1 illness and drug-addiction therapy can effectively suppress the heroin quitter's usual climax of the severe withdrawal reactions of the third and fourth days.

Observing, during the seven-day course of drug-addiction treatment, the total number of subjects with relieved withdrawal symptoms, their results, and their conditions.

Observing, After the XH-1 Health-Recovery Treatment the Rehabilitating Conditions of Heroin Users' Six Worst Item of Health Condition.

Heroin users' six worst items of health condition: 1. food appetite, 2. sleep, 3. spirited feel after awakening, 4. physical strength, 5. degree of comfort symptom, and 6. sexual appetite.

Observing each subject's daily condition of health-recovery treatment.

Observing the daily group population's changing tendency in terms of "good," "fair," and "poor" for each health item.

Observing the daily group population's changing tendency in terms of "good," "fair," and "poor" for the total health items.

Observing, after the seven-day health-recovery treatment, the rehabilitating effect of each health item.

Statistics of the effect of health-recovery treatment in percentage form.

Observing whether there are subjects with withdrawal symptoms during the course of health-recovery treatment.

During the Course of Health-Recovery treatment, It Is Necessary to Apply XH-1 Illness and Drug-Addiction Therapy to Treat Both Drug Induced or Non-Drug Induced Illnesses at the Same Time.

XH-1 treats the following twenty-one illnesses with conspicuous effects: 1. certain heart diseases, 2. high blood pressure, 3. low blood pressure, 4. headache, 5. migraine, 6. dizziness, 7. Menier's Syndrome, 8. glaucoma, 9. insomnia, 10. neck pain, 11. stiff neck, 12. allergic rhinitis, 13. sprain, 14. back pain and soreness, 15. joint pain, 16. arthredema, 17. stomach disorders, 18. dysmenorrhea, 19. shoulder periarthritis, 20. child neo-myopia, and 21. strange diseases of which the etiology is unknown.

When treating non-drug induced illnesses, it is necessary to list them individually into the statistics and observation.

Observing, When Heroin Quitters' Withdrawal Reacts, XH-1 Illnesses and Drug-Addiction Therapy's Relieving Conditions of the Seventeen Withdrawal Symptoms Produced.

Heroin quitters have the following seventeen withdrawal symptoms: 1) headache, 2) dizziness, 3) drowsiness, 4) yawning, 5) sneezing, 6) neck pain, 7) back and spinal pain, 8) lumbar pain, 9) muscle cramp of limbs, 10) abdominal pain, 11) cramp of internal organs, 12) nausea, 13) tight chest, 14) chest pain, 15) palpitation, 16) cold sweat with cold hands and feet, and 17) weakness.

Observing Each Subject's Daily Conditions of Drug-Addiction Treatment.

Everyday each heroin quitter who comes to receive XH-1 illness and drug-addiction therapy must fill out a "Statistical Chart of Each Subject's Daily Therapeutic Effect of Drug-addiction treatment" (Chart 1-A).

1. Observing, before receiving the daily XH-1 illness and drug-addiction therapy, heroin quitters' types of withdrawal symptoms by using three degrees, "heavy," "medium," and "light," to represent each withdrawal symptom's degree of severity.
2. Observing, after receiving the daily thirty minutes of XH-1 illness and drug-addiction treatment, the therapeutic effect of treating drug addiction and representing its degree with "conspicuously effective," "effective," and "not effective."
3. Increasing the frequency of a required urine test to observe and see if there are subjects going back to use the drug again, such as if a urine test shows drug positive, and list them as drug re-users and as the failure part of drug-addiction treatment.

Observing the Daily Total Condition of Drug-Addiction Treatment.

According to data "Statistical Chart of Each Subject's Daily Therapeutic Effect of Drug-Addiction treatment" (Chart 1-A), construct "Statistical Chart of the Daily Total Condition of Drug-Addiction treatment"(Chart 2), (2-1) to (2-7).

1. Observing, before receiving the daily XH-1 drug-addiction treatment, the total condition of the types of withdrawal symptoms, the degree of severity of the symptoms, and the group population changes of each

symptom. The degree of severity is represented by 3 levels: "heavy," "medium," and "light."
   2. Observing, after receiving the daily thirty minutes of drug-addiction treatment, the condition of the effects on the symptoms and its group population. The therapeutic effect on the symptoms is represented by three types of severity: "conspicuously effective," "effective," and "not effective."

Observing, during the Seven-Day Course of Drug-Addiction Treatment, XH-1 Therapeutic Effect on Each of the Seventeen Withdrawal Symptoms.

   1. According to data on "Group Population of the Daily Degree of Severity of Each Withdrawal Symptom" from data in the "Statistical Chart of the Daily Total Condition of Drug-Addiction Treatment" (Chart 2), construct "Graph of the Therapeutic Effect on Withdrawal Symptoms" (Chart 3), (3-1) to (3-15).
   2. Analyze each group population change curve of the daily degree of severity of each withdrawal symptom. Analyze the daily population of the degree of severity of each withdrawal symptom during the seven-day course of XH-1 drug-addiction treatment and its condition of daily increase, decrease, or elimination of the symptoms to assure XH-1's therapeutic effect on this withdrawal symptom.

Observing Whether the XH-1 Illness and Drug-Addiction Therapy Can Effectively Suppress the Heroin Quitter's Usual Climax of the Severe Withdrawal Reactions of the Third and Fourth Days.

Observing, during the course of drug-addiction treatment, whether each subject's daily average number of types of withdrawal symptoms has a tendency to increase or decrease, to assure whether XH-1 drug-addiction therapy can effectively suppress heroin quitter's usual climax of the severe withdrawal reaction of the third and fourth days.

   1. According to data from "Statistical Chart of the Daily Total Condition of Drug-Addiction Treatment" (Chart 2), statistically calculate: the group population of heroin quitters' daily total withdrawal symptoms.
   2. And then calculate: the daily average number of types of withdrawal symptoms per person.
   3. Construct "Graph of Daily Average Number of Types of Withdrawal Symptoms Per Person" (Chart 4).

Observing, during the course of drug-addiction treatment, whether the total group population change of the three degree types of severity of heroin addicts' withdrawal symptoms has a tendency to increase or decrease in order to assure whether XH-1 can effectively suppress heroin quitters' usual climax of the severe withdrawal reaction of the third and fourth days.

1. According to data from the "Statistical Chart of the Daily Total Condition of Drug-addiction Treatment" (Chart 2), statistically calculate: the total subjects' daily changes of the degree of severity of the symptoms.
2. Construct: "Graph of the Total Subjects' Daily Changes of the Degrees of Severity of Symptoms" (Chart 5).

Observing, during the seven-day course of drug-addiction treatment, the group population, condition, and relieving effect of the XH-1 illness and drug-addiction therapy on withdrawal symptoms.
Items to be analyzed and statistically calculated are:

1. Number of drug-addiction treatment participants.
2. Number of participants with the withdrawal symptoms relieved successfully.
3. Number of participants who failed.
4. Investigation and analysis for the reasons of failing.

Observing, after XH-1 Health-Recovery Treatment, the Rehabilitating Condition of Heroin Users' Six Worst Items of Health Condition.

Heroin Users' Six Worst Items of Health Condition: 1. food appetite, 2. sleep, 3. spirited feel after awakening, 4. physical strength, 5. degree of comfort symptom, and 6. sexual appetite.

Observing the Conditions of Each Subject's Daily Health-Recovery Treatment.

1. Everyday, each health-recovery treatment participant who comes to receive XH-1 therapy must fill out a "Statistical Chart of Each Subject's Daily Rehabilitating Degree" (Chart 1-B).
2. Observing the health condition of the six worst health items of subjects who received XH-1 health-recovery treatment daily and represent the health condition by "good," "fair," and "poor."
3. Increase the frequency of the required urine test to observe and see if

there are subjects going back to using drugs again; if the urine test shows drug positive, list them as drug re-users and as the failure part of drug-addiction treatment.

Analysis and Statistics of the Total Group Population of Daily Rehabilitating Degree of Health Items.

According to the data in the "Statistical Chart of Each Subject's Daily Rehabilitating Degree" (Chart 1-B), analyze and statistically calculate the daily total group population of rehabilitating degree of health items.

Construct "The Daily Statistical Chart of the Total Group Population's Rehabilitating Degree of Health Items" (Chart 6), (6-1) to (6-7).

Analysis and Statistics of Daily Group Population's Changing Tendency in Terms of Good, Fair, and Poor for Each Health Item.

According to data "The Daily Statistical Chart of the Total Group Population's Rehabilitating Degree of Health Items" (Chart 6), analyze and statistically calculate, during the seven-day course of health-recovery treatment using XH-1, each health item's group population's daily changing tendency in terms of "good," "fair," and "poor."

Construct "Graph of the Group Population's Daily Changing Tendency of Health Items in Terms of Good, Fair, and Poor" (Chart 7), (7-1) to (7-6).

Analyze and Statistically Calculate the Group Population's Daily Changing Tendency of Total Health Items in Terms of Good, Fair, and Poor.

According to data "The Daily Statistical Chart of the Total Group Population's Rehabilitating Degree of Health Items" (Chart 6), analyze and statistically calculate, during the seven-day course of health-recovery treatment using XH-1, the total group population's daily changing tendency of the total health items in terms of "good," "fair," and "poor."

Construct "Graph of Total Group Population's Daily Changing Tendency of the Total Health Items in Terms of Good, Fair, and Poor" (Chart 8).

Analysis and Statistics of the Rehabilitation Results of Each Health Item on the Seventh Day.

According to data in "The Daily Statistical Chart of the Total Group Population's Rehabilitating Degree of Health Items" (Chart 6), analyze and statistically calculate, after the seven-day course of health-recovery treatment, XH-1's rehabilitating effect on heroin users' each of the six worst items of health condition on the last day (seventh day) calculated by the group population in terms of "good," "fair," and "poor."

Analysis and Statistics of Effects of Rehabilitation Treatment.

According to data in "The Daily Statistical Chart of the Total Group Population's Rehabilitating Degree of Health Items" (Chart 6), analyze and statistically calculate, after the seven-day course of health-recovery treatment, XH-1's total rehabilitation effect on heroin users' six worst items of health condition on the last day (seventh day) in percentage form of those who really participated in the health-recovery treatment.

Observing Whether There Are Subjects With Withdrawal Symptoms During the Seven-Day Course of Health-Recovery Treatment.

1. Construct "Statistical Chart of the Group Population's Daily Number of Types of Withdrawal Symptoms During the Course of Health-Recovery Treatment" (Chart 9).
2. If there are subjects with withdrawal symptoms, calculate them as the failed part of drug-addiction treatment.

During the Course of Health-Recovery Treatment, It Is Necessary to Apply XH-1 Illness and Drug-Addiction Therapy to Treat Both Drug Induced or Non-Drug Induced Illnesses at the Same Time.

XH-1 Has Conspicuous Therapeutic Effects on Twenty-one Types of Illnesses:

1. certain heart diseases, 2. high blood pressure, 3. low blood pressure, 4. headache, 5. migraine, 6. dizziness, 7. Menier's Syndrome, 8. glaucoma, 9. insomnia, 10. neck pain, 11. stiff neck, 12. allergic rhinitis, 13. sprain, 14. back pain and soreness, 15. joint pain, 16. arthredema, 17. stomach disorders, 18. dysmenorrhea, 19. shoulder periarthritis, 20. child neo-myopia, and 21. strange diseases of which the etiology is unknown.

When treating non-drug induced illnesses, each of them must be listed individually into the statistics and observation at the same time.

Reference Therapeutic Locations for the Twenty-one Types of Illnesses

	location	location	
1. certain heart diseases	N	Z	
(For emergency rescue, add:)	J		painful/tight chest point(s)
2. high blood pressure	N	Q	discomfortpoint(s)
3. low blood pressure	N	Q	discomfort point(s)
4. headache	N		headache point(s)
5. migraine	N		headache point(s)
6. dizziness	N	Y	discomfort point(s)
7. Menier's Syndrome	N	G	discomfort point(s)
8. glaucoma	N	M	discomfort point(s)
9. insomnia	N	Z	
10. neck pain			painful point(s)
11. stiff neck			painful point(s)
12. allergic rhinitis		B	
13. sprain			painful point(s)
14. back pain and soreness			painful/sore point(s)
15. joint pain			painful point(s)
16. arthredema			edema point(s)
17. stomach disorders		Z	discomfort point(s)
18. dysmenorrhea		S	painful point(s)
19. shoulder periarthritis			painful point(s)
20. child neo-myopia		M	
21. strange diseases of which the etiology is unknown			painful discomfort point(s)

Location B: At the highest point of the nasolabial groove.
Location J: On the lower portion of the cervical vertebrae.
Location M: Immediately superior to the inner canthus.
Location N: Three fingers' breadth above the transverse crease of the wrist, between the tendons of m. palmaris longus and m. flexor radialis.
Location Q: When the elbow is flexed, the point is in the depression at the lateral end of the transverse cubital crease.
Location S: Four fingers' breadth directly above the tip of the medial malleolus, on the posterior border of the medial aspect of the tibia.
Location G: Immediately anterior to the tragus.
Location Y: Slightly above the midway between the medial ends of the two eyebrows.
Location Z: When the knee is flexed, four fingers' breadth below the lower border of the patella, one finger breadth from the anterior crest of the tibia, in m. tibialis anterior.

For photographic illustration of the therapeutic locations, see PP. 136 & 137.

It is a must to relieve drug quitters' non-drug induced illnesses and pains; otherwise, due to the existence of the illnesses and pain which need to be solved, drug quitters would continue to take drugs. When treating the non-drug induced illnesses, they must be listed individually into the statistics and be observed at the same time.

Therapeutic Locations for the Course of Drug-Addiction Treatment and the Course of Health-Recovery Treatment.

1. Course of drug-addiction treatment: once per day, thirty minutes each time, total of seven days.
   Therapeutic locations:
   Location J pairs with Location N
   Location Z pairs with Location N (or the skin surface of painful/ discomfort points)
2. Course of health-recovery treatment: once per day, thirty minutes each time, total of seven days.
   Therapeutic locations:
   Location J pairs with Location N
   Location Z pairs with Location S

Rules for the Usage of XH-1 Rehabilitation Therapeutic Machine.

1. Place the XH-1 electrodes on the drug quitters' skin surface of the related and painful/discomfort locations.
2. There are three types of electrode lines-blue, yellow, and green:
   Blue line is a small electrical-current line.
   Yellow line is a weak, small electrical-current line.
   Green line is the weakest small electrical-current line.
   a. Use blue line for treating various locations on the body and limbs, e.g., certain heart diseases, neck pain, stiff neck, sprain, lumbar pain/soreness, joint pain, arthredema, stomach disorders, dysmenorrhea, and shoulder periarthritis, and for treating high blood pressure and low blood pressure on locations N and Q. (See photographic illustration on lower page 128, right side of page 132, and upper page 134.)
   b. Use yellow line for treating locations on the head area, e.g., headache, migraine, dizziness, Menier's Syndrome, and allergic rhinitis. (See photographic illustration on lower page 130 and upper page 133.)
   c. Use green line for treating locations around the eye area, e.g., glaucoma and child neo-myopia. (See photographic illustration on upper and lower page 123.)
3. Between the skin surface and the electrodes, fill in a 1.2 cm. area of tap-water moistened eight-layer paper towel for isolation. The purpose of isolation is to prevent skin contamination. Dispose of the paper towel after use.
4. There is no positive or negative difference between the electrodes.
5. Use household tapes to hold the electrodes.
6. Control the output dial to the extent so that the drug quitter feels comfortable.

The Electrical Performance of the XH-1 Rehabilitation Therapeutic Machine.

What the XH-1 rehabilitation therapeutic machine sends out is a natural human wave. The time-length of each wave is a few milliseconds long, and at approximately one pulse per second. The electrical current output is 0.002 milliamp, at the rate of 0.003 milliwatt. If using two AA dry batteries, DC three volt, every day at two hours per day, the machine can run for one year and two months, so it is extremely frugal on electrical consumption. Due to the fact that the XH-1 rehabilitation therapeutic machine works at the state of weak electrical current and small rate of consumption, it is very safe.

However, using the batteries for a long time can cause the output wave form to change and, hence, affects the therapeutic effect. Therefore it is recommended to use AC as a power source, because the XH-1 rehabilitation therapeutic machine can convert 120 volt or 220 volt of an AC power source into an extremely stable DC 2.4 volt, allow the output wave shape to stabilize and not change, and raise the therapeutic effect.

NOTE:
1. According to the U.S. standard, more than 15 milliamp of electrical current passing through the human heart is considered dangerous. Lower than 1 milliamp is considered completely safe.
2. Other pulse therapeutic machines produced in the U.S. and Japan have an electrical current between 30 milliamp to 100 milliamp, which way exceeds the lower-than-1 milliamp electrical current value.

U.S. Expert's Test Report on XH-1 Rehabilitation Therapeutic Machine

10-13-93

The performance characteristics of the XH-1 Rehabilitation machine were tested by Lewis C. Ensor Company. Mr. Ensor's prior experience includes 35 years of engineering research and development of electronic transducers of many types at the National Bureau of Standards (now National Institute of Standards and Technology) in Washington, D.C. and as Senior Project Engineer and later as a Consultant at Endevco Corporation (now a division of Meggit Corporation, United Kingdom) at San Juan Capistrano, CA 92675. Many of the years of experience envolved the calibration and evaluation of transducers and associated electronics of similar characteristics to the XH-1 machine.

TABLE: OUTPUT VERSUS RESISTIVE LOAD

LOAD OHMS	CABLE COLOR	FREQUENCY PULSES/SEC	AVERAGE MILLIAMPS	AVERAGE MILLIWATTS
10000	Blue	0.9	0.18	0.32
10000	Yellow	0.9	0.14	0.20
10000	Green	0.9	0.02	0.0044
1000000	Blue	0.9	0.002	0.003

The 1,000,000 ohm test is typical for the resistance of the human body. The average current is very low and safe when applied to the human body.

Dangerous current levels are those above about 15 milliamps but below 1 millamp is considered completely safe according to the Federal Engineering Department associated with the National Electric Code and according to the State of California OSHA Consultation Group. The average current levels for this XH-1 machine are less than 1/5 of a milliamp and are therefore totally safe and easily tolerated for treatment.

Lewis C. Ensor Company

Lewis C. Ensor
Post Office Box 1865
Tustin, CA 92681, U.S.A.

Document No. 2001/235   (Translation)

**RESULTS AND PROOF OF USING THE
XH ONE THERAPEUTIC MACHINE
FOR TREATING ILLNESS AND DRUG ADDICTION**

DEPARTMENT OF HEALTH,
BANGKOK METROPOLITAN
January 21, 1991

DOCUMENT SEND TO: DR. YAN LAIYIN

The XH One therapeutic machine, which was invented and created by the disease and drug treating expert--Dr, Yan Laiyin, uses a small electric current to treat illnesses and drug addiction, and able to achieve very good and conspicuous results. It is very suitable for emergency rescuing the severe and dangerous drug withdrawal syndrome of heroine addicts.

According to Bangkok Metropolitan government's approval, for 4 years using the XH One therapeutic machine to treat illness and drug addiction in the 12th Narcotic Clinic, there has been no adverse effects found, its safety is trustworthy, and the effectiveness is conspicuous.   For treating illness and drug addiction, its efficacy is no less than 90%.

Kachit Choopanya
Administration of
Health department

24

ที่ กท. 2001/ 235

สำนักอนามัย กรุงเทพมหานคร

173 ถนนดินสอ เสาชิงช้า กท 10200

วันที่ 21 มกราคม 2534

เรื่อง แจ้งผลการรักษาโรค ถอนพิษยาเสพติดด้วยเครื่อง XII

เรียน Dr. Yan Lai Yin

ตามที่ท่าน Dr. Yan Lai Yin เป็นผู้เชี่ยวชาญการรักษาโรค ถอนพิษยาเสพติด และเป็นผู้คิดค้น-ผลิตเครื่องมือ XII ซึ่งมีสมรรถนะของคลื่นกำลังภายในตัวยานั้น เมื่อนำไปใช้ในการรักษาโรคถอนพิษยาเสพติดได้ผลดีเห็นได้อย่างชัดเจนภายใน 5-15 นาที จึงมีความเหมาะสมอย่างยิ่งที่จะใช้ในการช่วยชีวิตและขจัดอาการอันตรายอันเกิดจากอาการเสี้ยนยาของผู้ติดยาเสพติดเฮโรอีน

ตามที่ทางราชการกรุงเทพมหานครได้ใช้เครื่องมือคลื่นกำลังภายใน XH นี้ให้บริการรักษาโรคถอนพิษยาเสพติด ณ. คลินิกยาเสพติดที่ 12 เป็นเวลา 4 ปีมานี้ไม่เคยปรากฏเหตุการณ์ในทางที่ไม่ดี แต่เป็นการรักษาที่ปลอดภัยเป็นที่น่าไว้วางใจได้ และได้ผลดีเห็นได้อย่างเด่นชัด ไม่ต่ำกว่า 90%.

จึงเรียนมาเพื่อทราบ และขอบคุณอย่างยิ่งที่ให้ความร่วมมือ.

XH型信息治療儀
用於治病戒毒結果

曼谷市衛生處

文件送到：Dr. Yan Laiyin 晏萊蔭醫師

　　治病、戒毒專家 Dr. Yan Laiyin 晏萊蔭醫師，所發明創造的XH型信息治療儀，輸出模仿人體的氣功電磁波，用於治病戒毒，能在五至十五分鐘之內，得到很明顯很好的效果。非常適合搶救，消除戒海洛英者、毒癮嚴重發作時的危象。

　　經曼谷市政府批准，用XH信息治療儀，治病、戒毒在第十二治病戒毒所，四年來，沒有發現不好的情況，安全可相信，療效明顯。用於治病、戒毒，效果不會少於９０％。

ขอแสดงความนับถือ

曼谷市第十二治病戒毒所翻譯

สำนักเลขานุการ

โทร. 224-4680

ที่ กท. 2001/๒๓๕

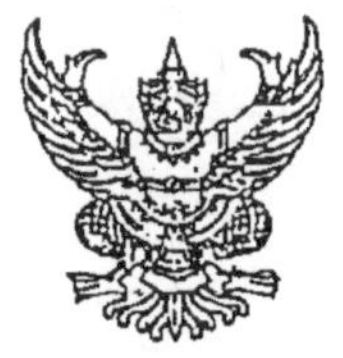

สำนักอนามัย กรุงเทพมหานคร

173 ถนนดินสอ เสาชิงช้า กท 10200

วันที่ 21 มกราคม 2534

เรื่อง แจ้งผลการรักษาโรค ถอนพิษยาเสพติดด้วยเครื่อง XH

เรียน Dr. Yan Lai Yin

ตามที่ท่าน   Dr. Yan Lai Yin   เป็นผู้เชี่ยวชาญการรักษาโรค ถอนพิษยาเสพติด และเป็นผู้คิดค้น-ผลิตเครื่องมือ XH   ซึ่งมีสมรรถนะของคลื่นกำลังภายในด้วยนั้น เมื่อนำไปใช้ในการรักษาโรคถอนพิษยาเสพติดได้ผลดีเห็นได้อย่างชัดเจนภายใน 5-15 นาที จึงมีความเหมาะสมอย่างยิ่งที่จะใช้ในการช่วยชีวิตและขจัดอาการอันตรายอันเกิดจากอาการเสี่ยงยาของผู้ติดยาเสพติดเฮโรอีน

ตามที่ทางราชการกรุงเทพมหานครได้ใช้เครื่องมือคลื่นกำลังภายใน XH นี้ให้บริการรักษาโรคถอนพิษยาเสพติด ณ. คลินิกยาเสพติดที่ 12 เป็นเวลา 4 ปีมานี้ไม่เคยปรากฏเหตุการณ์ในทางที่ไม่ดี แต่เป็นการรักษาที่ปลอดภัยเป็นที่น่าไว้วางใจได้ และได้ผลดีเห็นได้อย่างเด่นชัด ไม่ต่ำกว่า 90%.

จึงเรียนมาเพื่อทราบ และขอบคุณอย่างยิ่งที่ให้ความร่วมมือ.

ขอแสดงความนับถือ

(นายขจิต ชูบัญญา)
รองผู้อำนวยการสำนักอนามัย

สำนักเลขานุการ

โทร. 224-4680

26

INTRODUCING THE XH THERAPY
BY THE 12TH NARCOTIC CLINIC
(19TH MEDICAL CLINIC)

CLINICALLY OBSERVED BY
SUNEEPORN ANUTTARAKULVANICH,
PERSON IN CHARGE OF
THE DRUG ADDICTION TREATING DEPARTMENT, THAILAND
NOVEMBER 2, 1989

According to the patients, the XH therapy has miraculous effect on treating heart diseases, high blood pressure, and drug addiction, including the illnesses that are drug induced or non-drug induced.

The letters "XH" of the XH therapy stands for the Chinese characters which mean to "relieve illness and pain" and "rehabilitating health".

The XH therapy is made of two parts:
1. Dr. Yan Laiyin's specialized medical technic.
2. The therapeutic machine, which was invented by Dr. Yan Laiyin and able to treat illnesses without the use of medication.

The XH therapy is used for treating drug addiction, including the following 4 contents:

1. Drug addiction treatment.
2. Relieve the withdrawal symptoms.
3. Treat drug induced or non-drug induced illnesses and pain.
4. Rehabilitating to normal health.

INTRODUCTION:

1. XH therapy can rehabilitate various parts of the bodily functions to healthy level. In 7 days, XH therapy is able to relieve the illnesses and dangers of withdrawal syndrome; hence distinguish patients' need to take drugs, therefore, achieve the goal of quitting drug.

2. In 15 to 30 minutes, XH therapy is able to relieve illnesses,
including those that are due to drug withdrawal.
There are 17 illnesses due to heroin withdrawal:

     1. headache 2. dizziness 3. drowsiness 4. yawning
     5. sneezing 6. neck pain 7. back and spinal pain
     8. lumbar pain 9. muscle cramp of limbs 10. abdominal
     pain 11. pain and cramp of internal organs 12. nausea
     13. tight chest 14. chest pain 15. palpitation
     16. cold sweat and hands/feet 17. weakness.

3. There are 20 illnesses XH therapy can treat:

     1. certain heart diseases 2. high blood pressure 3.
     low blood pressure 4. headache 5. migraine
     6. dizziness 7. sea sick 8. insomnia 9. neck pain
     10. stiff neck 11. rhinitis 12. cold 13. sprain
     14. pain in joints 15. asthma 16. numbness of the
     limbs 17. swollen joints 18. stomach disorders
     19. nausea 20. dysmenorrhea.

4. Rehabilitate health.

     Within a short period of time, the XH therapy can relieve
the illness secondary to drug withdrawal, able to make the heart,
blood pressure, nervous system, and other functions of the body
return to normal level. After 7 days of drug addiction treatment
and another 7 days of rehabilitation treatment, most of the drug
quitters are back to normal health level and able to live and
work like normal people.

     3 years of experience with XH therapy for treating drug
addiction has proved the following:

     1. Patients who are highly motivated to quit drugs can
     see conspicuous results in 5 to 7 days, no longer take
     drugs, and do not have the pain and suffering due to
     drug withdrawal syndrome.

     2.   It takes only 5 to 15 minutes of XH treatment to
     relieve patients' pain and suffering of the drug
     withdrawal syndrome. When we serve the patients with
     XH therapy, it takes one 15 minute treatment each day
     on the patient, and very good results have been proven.

     3. The results show that by using the XH therapy to
     treat illnesses, whether they are drug induced or non-
     drug induced, it takes 7 days of treatment to relieve
     them in most cases.

4. By using the XH therapy to rehabilitate health, the
drug addicts experience conspicuous improvements after
the treatment. Patients have good appetites and eat
well, good sleep, relief from cramps during sleep,
enhanced sexual function, resolution from dizziness,
and enhanced body energy. What used to be agonizing to
wake up and having difficulty to get off the bed, after
the treatment, became easy to get off the bed after
awakening, feels comfortable, energetic, and able to
handle normal work.

<u>CONCLUSION:</u>

By using the XH therapy to treat drug addiction, the
patients can be relieved of the pain and agony of the drug
withdrawal syndrome, and by using the treatment for illnesses to
rehabilitate to normal health, the results show more than 95%
efficacy. The realistic results proved that the figure is even
higher than Dr. Yan's initial estimate of 85% efficacy.

When Dr. Yan Laiyin treats drug addiction, he is very much
aware of the drug quitters' illnesses, whether they are drug
induced or non-drug induced, and treats the illnesses and drug
addiction together with the same time. This therapy achieved
very good results for quitting drug.

After the clinical observation, XH therapy is not just for
treating drug addiction, but also for treating other illnesses.
This therapy can bring Thailand huge benefit. In order to let
the Thai people receive the XH therapy, I like to especially
suggest:

1.   We should make the XH therapy remain in Thailand, and have
the inventor and medical expert, Dr. Yan Laiyin, spread
instructions.

2. We should use this therapy to set up a new medical department
and apply this medication-free illness-treating XH therapy to
expand the medicine of Thailand.

If the related departments can achieve this goal
successfully, then Thailand can benefit greatly by... 1. Reduce
a huge amount of medical cost. e.g. Just the amount of money
saved on pain killers is tremendous. 2.   Able to help the
citizens to become healthy, so a large amount of medication for
treating illnesses can be eliminated, avoid the danger of other
illnesses associated with taking medication, and greatly
strengthen the citizens' health standards.

TRANSLATED BY
Peter Shieh

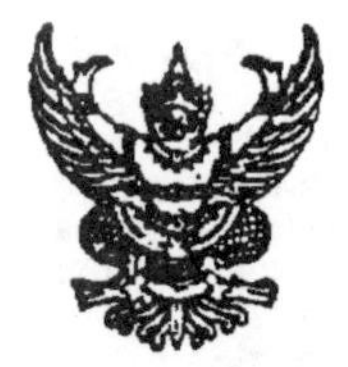

第 十 二 戒 毒 醫 務 所
第 十 九 醫 務 所
介 紹「消」醫 法
由 素 尼 蓬 參 加 臨 床 觀 察
一 九 八 九 年 十 一 月 二 日

　　根據病人說：「消」醫法，對醫治心臟病、高血壓、解毒，包括消除吸毒引起的及非吸毒引起的各種病痛，能取得神奇的效果。

　　「消」醫法，「消」是指能減輕或消除病痛的意思。

　　「消」醫法是由兩部份組成：

一、晏萊蓬醫師的專門醫術。

二、晏萊蓬醫師發明的醫病機器，用在醫病，不用吃藥。

　　「消」醫法用於解毒，包括四項內容：

一、解戒毒。

二、消除吸毒者的痛苦。

三、治療吸毒引起的及非吸毒引起的病。

四、康復治療，恢復身體健康。

　　介紹：

一、「消」醫法，能恢復身體各部份的功能，使身體健康起來，在七天之內，就能消除因缺毒所引起的痛苦及危險，使病人得以不用再吸毒，而達到解毒、戒毒的目的。

二、「消」醫法，能在十五分鐘至卅分鐘內，減輕或消除病痛，包括毒癮發作所引起的痛苦。

　　毒癮發作引起的痛苦共計有十七種。

　　1.頭痛 2.頭暈 3.欲睡 4.打哈欠 5.打噴嚏 6.頸痛 7.背脊痛 8.腰痛 9.手腳肌肉痙攣痛 10.肚痠 11.內臟痙攣痛 12.嘔吐 13.胸悶 14.胸痛 15.心悸心速 16.手腳冷 17.無力。

三.「消」醫法可醫治廿種病

　　1. 心臟病 2. 高血壓 3. 低血壓 4. 頭痛 5. 偏頭痛 6. 頭暈 7. 暈車船 8. 失眠 9. 頸痛 10. 落枕 11. 鼻炎 12. 感冒 13. 扭傷 14. 關節痛 15. 哮喘 16. 手腳麻 17. 關節腫 18. 胃病 19. 嘔吐 20. 月經痛

四 恢復身體健康

　　「消」醫法，能在極短的時間內，減輕或消除吸毒者的痛苦，使心臟、血壓、神經及身體各部份的功能，恢復正常起來，吸毒者經解毒治療七天，再經康復治療七天，大部份吸毒者身體能健康起來，能如正常人那樣生活工作。

　　三年的經驗證明了「消」醫法用於解毒戒毒。

一、大部份病人「指有心要戒毒者」五天至七天內，就能明顯見到戒毒的效果。不再吸毒，也不會發生缺毒引起的痛苦。

二、吸毒者毒癮發作引起的痛苦，用「消」醫法治療，五至十五分鐘就可減輕或消除。

　　根據「消」醫法的解（戒）毒規定，吸毒者如能住入醫院，用「消」醫法解毒，一天三次，每次十五分鐘，不用服藥，就能得到好的解毒戒毒效果。但是現在我們服務病人，僅每天一次，每次十五分鐘，實際證明也得到比較好的效果。

三、「消」醫法用於治病的效果，無論是吸毒引起的病，或非吸毒引起的病，經過十天的治療，大部份能逐漸好轉或消除。

四、用「消」醫法恢復身體健康，吸毒者經治療都能取得明顯的療效，病人想吃，吃得多，睡得好，睡眠時抽筋的現象減少或消除。性功能增強，頭暈現象減輕或消除，體力增強。病人原來睡後醒來，感到人很痛苦，難以起床，經治療，每天睡醒後能立即起來，自我感覺舒服，精力旺盛，並能勝任正常工作。

結　語：

　　「消」醫法用於解毒，能減輕或消除因不再吸毒而因毒癮發作所引起的痛苦，用於治病，恢復身體健康，都能取得九十五％以上的好效果，實際療效證明超過了晏萊薩醫師肯定的八十五％的效果。

　　晏萊薩醫師在解毒時，非常注意吸毒者身上的病，無論是吸毒引起的，或非吸毒引起的，結合解毒一起，同時給予治療，這個辦法，使解毒取得非常好的效果。

通過臨床治療觀察，「消」醫法不僅可用於解毒，也可用於治療其他疾病，這個醫法能給泰國帶來很大利益，爲使泰國人民得到這個「消」醫法，特建議：

一、應該把這「消」醫法留在泰國，由發明人、醫學專家 DR. YAN LAIYIN 晏萊蔭醫師傳授。

二、應用這個醫法成立一個新的醫學部門，「治病不用藥」使泰國醫學發展起來。

有關部門如能把這項目落實成功，將使泰國得到利益多多……。1. 減少大量大量的醫藥費。如：僅減少止痛藥這一項就了不得了。2. 能幫助人民身體健康起來，使病人免除爲治病而服用大量藥物，免除因服藥而引起其他疾病的危險性，可大大地增強人民健康的水準。

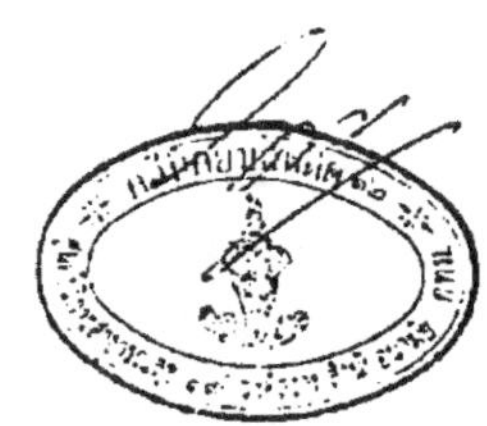

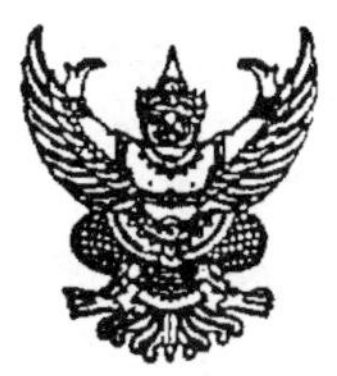

คลีนิคยาเสพติด 12   ศูนย์บริการสาธารณสุข 19 วงศ์สว่าง

แนะนำการบำบัดรักษา

ด้วย

วิธี   เขียว

โดย.   สุณิภรณ์ อนุกกรกุลวนิช

ผู้ร่วมปฏิบัติการ และสังเกตุการณ์

วันที่ 2 พฤศจิกายน 2532

33

การรักษา ... ผู้ป่วยเกี่ยวกับการบำบัดรักษาวิธี เวียว ซึ่งใช้ในการรักษา โรคหัวใจ
โรคความดันโลหิต การบำบัดรักษาภูมิแพ้นานาเสพติด ตลอดจนการจัดการทุกข์ทรมานอันเนื่องมาจาก
โรคต่าง ๆ โดยละคี คลายปัญหาริ

<u>และนำการบำบัดรักษาวิธี เวียว</u>

เวียว หมายถึง การขจัดการทุกข์ทรมานอันเนื่องมาจากโรคต่าง ๆ ในตลอด พร้อมหายไป
<u>การบำบัดรักษาวิธี เวียว นี้ประกอบควบความสำคัญเป็น 2 ส่วน รวมกันดังนี้</u>

ความสำคัญส่วนที่ 1 คือ เทคนิคและวิธีการบำบัดรักษาอย่างชำนาญและเขียวชาญของ DR.
yan Laiyin

ความสำคัญส่วนที่ 2 คือ เครื่องมือที่ DR. yan Laiyin ค้นหาวาไว้มาใช้ในการรักษาโรค
ต่าง ๆ โดยไม่ต้องใช้ยา

ต่อไปนี้ จะกล่าวถึงการบำบัดรักษาวิธี เวียว ซึ่งใช้ในการบำบัดรักษาคนติดยา เสพติดโดย
มุ่งเนนเบี้องสาระสำคัญ 4 ประการควยกันคือ

1 ถอนพิษยา

2 ขจัดอาการทรมานอันเนื่องมาจากยาเสพติด

3 บำบัดรักษาโรคทางกายต่าง ๆ ทั้งที่เนื่องมาจากยาเสพติด และที่ไม่ใช่เนื่องมาจากยาเสพติด

4 ฟื้นฟูสุขภาพให้แข็งแรงขึ้น

<u>อริบาย</u>

1. การบำบัดรักษาวิธี เวียว นี้ สามารถปรับเสริมการทำงานของระบบควัยวะต่าง ๆ ของ
ร่างกายให้ทำงานแรงแรงขึ้น เพื่อร่างกายจะไปขับความสามารถ ขจัดพิษของสิ่งเสพติดออกมาโดยอย่างมี
ประสิทธิภาพขึ้น ซึ่งจะอยู่ในระยะเวราประมาณ 7 วัน ผู้ป่วยสามารถอยู่ยา ๆ โดยไม่ต้องทุกข์ทรมานอัน
เนื่องมาจากการวาดยา และไม่มีอันตรายใด ๆ ทำให้ผู้ป่วยไม่กำเป็นของไขยาเสพติดอีก

2. สามารถใช้วิธี เวียว นี้ ระยะเฉลาเรียง 15 – 30 นาที กระดพริ้ขจัดอาการทุกข์
ทรมานของผู้ป่วยได้ รวมทั้งอาการทุกข์ทรมานอันเกิดจากการ<u>วาดยา</u>ของผู้ติดยาเสพติด ซึ่งอาคกล่าวไว้
ประมาณ 17 อาการ ดังนี้

1 ปวดศีรษะ	9 ปวดตามเนื้อแขนขาและกระดูก
2 มึน วิงเวียนศีรษะ	10 ปวดหรง
3 ง่วง	11 อาการ ปวด เกร็งและกระตุกในขา
4 ราว	12 อาเจียน
5 ราม	13 แน่นหน้าอก
6 ปวดกันคอ	14 เจ็บหน้าอก
7 ปวดหลัง	15 หัวใจเต้นเร็ว
8 ปวดเอว	16 มือ เท้า เย็น
	17 ไข้ขึ้นสูง – ตอนเช้า

34

ผู้ที่ใช้ครักษาแบบ เซียวนี้ ใช้สามารถรักษาโรคนี้ ๆ ได้ ๒ ๒ วิธี ดังนี้

1 โรคหัวใจ	11 ไซนัส
2 ความดันโลหิตสูง	12 หวัด
3 ความดันโลหิตต่ำ	13 เหลูจัดยาก
4 ปวดศีรษะ	14 ปวดคอ
5 ปวดศีรษะข้างเดียว	15 หอบ หืด
6 มึน วิงเวียนศีรษะ	16 แขน ราา
7 เมารถ เมาเรือ	17 ออนวม
8 นอนไม่หลับ	18 โรคกะเพาะอาหาร
9 ปวดคนคอ	19 กาเจียน
10 กกหมอน	20 ปวดประจำเดือน

4. การฟื้นคืนสุขภาพให้แข็งแรงขึ้น วิธีการบำบัดรักษาแบบ เซียวนี้ สามารถลดหรือจัดอาการ
ทุกส่วนานส่วนใหญ่ของผู้ป่วยยาเสพติดได้ในเวลาอันสั้นแลว บังทำให้ระบบการทำงานของหัวใจ ความดัน
ระบบประสาท และระบบอื่น ๆ ของร่างกายให้ฟื้นคืนสุขภาพแข็งแรงขึ้น ซึ่งปกติแลวผู้ป่วยที่ผ่านการบำบัด
รักษาถอนพิษยา 7 วัน และควรได้รับการบำบัดให้ฟื้นคืนสุขภาพอีก 7 วัน ผู้ป่วยส่วนใหญ่จะมีสุขภาพที่แข็งแรง
ขึ้น และสามารถมีชีวิตการเป็นอยู่อย่างปกติได้

<u>จากประสพการณ์ 5 ปี</u> ที่ผ่านมาได้มีการใช้การบำบัดรักษาแบบ เซียวนี้ ในการบำบัดรักษาถอน
พิษยาเสพติด ได้ประจักษ์ความจริงยืนยันได้ว่า

1 ผู้ป่วยส่วนใหญ่ (หากที่มีความทั้งใจระยะเลิกยาเสพติดสำเร็จได้ใน 5 – 7 วัน) จะประจักษ์ยืน
ของการถอนพิษยา แม้ไม่เสพยาเสพติดก็ตาม จะยังไม่มีอาการทรมาน

2 อาการทุกทรมานกันเกิดจากการรักษาของผู้ติดยาเสพติด เมื่อได้ใช้วิธี เซียวนี้ ในระยะ
เวลาเพียง 5 – 15 นาที ก็สามารถลดหรือจัดอาการทรมานได้ ซึ่งตามทฤษฎีการบำบัดรักษาถอนพิษยา
เสพติด ควยวิธีนี้ ผู้ป่วยติดยาเสพติดเมื่อเข้ารับการรักษาตัวไปสถานพยาบาล โดยรับการบำบัดรักษา
วันละ 3 ครั้ง ครั้งละ 15 นาที โดยไม่ต้องใช้ยา จะได้ผลดี แต่ในปัจจุบันนี้ ได้มีการให้บริการแกผู้ป่วย
มาก เพียงวันละ 1 ครั้ง ๆ ละ 15 นาที ก็โดยลดพิษกัน

3 ผลกัดโรคในผู้ป่วย ไม่ว่าจะเป็นโรคที่เนื่องมาจากยาเสพติดหรือโดโรคทาง เมื่อได้รับการ
บำบัดแบบ เซียวนี้แลว ประมาณ 10 กว่าวัน จะมีการเปลี่ยนแปลงที่ดีขึ้นเรื่อย ๆ หรือหายจากโรคนั้น ๆ
ได้ และจากการที่พบเห็นมานี้ ไม่เพียงแต่จะรักษาโรค 20 โรคตามที่ DR. YAN LAIYIN
ได้เคยยกไว้ดังกล่าวข้างกันเท่านั้นยังมีโรคริกมากมายที่รักษาโดยดี เช่น โรคไหล่ลามทุ่ง โรคมานชำ
สมรรถภาพทางเพศ ปวดศีรษะรันเนื่องมาจากลายตาบีความดันบิดปกติ และโรคต่าง ๆ ที่ทางโรงพยาบาล
หรือแพทย์แผนปัจจุบันกรวจหาไม่พบสาเหตุ เมื่อได้รับการบำบัดรักษาก็โดยดีเนียม

35

การบำบัดรักษาถอนพิษยา เข้าวันนั้น ผู้ป่วยจะได้รับการบำบัดรักษา จะมีการเปลี่ยน
แปลงที่ดีขึ้น คือทำให้กอยากรับประทานอาหาร รับประทานอาหารได้ มากขึ้น นอนหลับได้ดีขึ้น อาการ
กระตุก (เพ้าคลั่ง) จะลดน้อยลงจนหายกระตุก ผู้ป่วยส่วนใหญ่บอกว่ามีเรี่ยวแรงทางเพศดีขึ้น เนื้อตัวแข็ง
แรงและอุ่นขึ้นมีกำลังการทำงานได้ดี อาการหาวเรอมีน้ำตาไหลดีขึ้น ทดลองเนื้อตัวอุ่นขึ้น หลังก็มีแรงอนกระตุกขึ้นได้อย่างรวด
เร็วและอุ่นยาวนาน (เพราะเนื้อตัวคนที่ยังไม่ได้รับการบำบัดรักษาแบบ เร็ววันนี้ หนังเนื้อคนกว่าจะอุ่นขึ้นจาก
ที่เย็นได้ ดังนั้นใจมากและนานจะต้องและกันขึ้นให้คนสามารถมีกำลังกาย กำลังใจในการประกอบอาชีพได้

สรุป

จากการที่ได้ใช้วิธีการบำบัดรักษาถอนพิษยา แบบเจี๋ยวในการบำบัดรักษาผู้ติดยาเสพติดนั้น
ความสามารถในการแพทย์หรือจัดการการทุกขทรมาน การบำบัดรักษาโรคต่าง ๆ การคืนสุขภาพไทยดี
ไม่น้อยกว่า 95 % ซึ่งไทยมมากกว่าที่ DR. YAN LAIYIN เคยบอกไว้ประมาณ 85% เรียกว่า

ในการบำบัดรักษาถอนพิษยาเสพติดของ DR. YAN LAIYIN นั้นท่านเนกามชนการบำบัดรักษา
โรคต่าง ๆ ซึ่งอยู่ในร่างกายผู้ป่วยหรือยไม่ว่าโรคนั้น ๆ จะเป็นโรคที่เนื่องมาจากยาเสพติด หรือมิใช่ยา
เสพติดก็ตาม ควบรู้ไปกับการถอนพิษยา และสิ่งนี้เองที่เป็นจุดอย่างยิ่งสิ่งหนึ่ง ที่ทำให้นิการบำบัดรักษาถอน
พิษยาเสพติดไทยดี

<u>ข้อเสนอแนะ</u>

จากการที่เผยแพร่การรักษาประจัดขนี้ความจริงแล้วนี้ ไม่เพียงแต่จะบำบัดรักษาถอนพิษยาเสพติด
เท่านั้นการใช้ในการบำบัดโรคอื่น ๆ ได้รับจะเกิดประโยชน์ต่อประชาชนชาวไทย และประเทศชาติเป็นอย่าง
จึงมีความจำเป็นและขอเสนอแนะดังนี้

1 ควรจะนำให้วิธีการรักษา แบบนี้มีไว้ในเบื้องไทยเหตุที่จะขณะนี้ เรามีอาการอ่อนว่ารักที่จะ
ถ่ายออกง่ายแล้วนี้

2 น่าที่จะนำเราสู่วงการแพทย์ของเรา และคนละว่าในเจริญการพนาขึ่ง รืนไป
หากผานผู้มีอำนาจ หน้าที่ได้ดำเนินการสำเร็จเราก็เกิดผลต่อคุณประโยชน์ให้ประเทศชาติมากมาย คือ

1 ประเทศชาติจะประหยัดค่ายาไทยอย่างมากหลาย แห่งประหยัดยาแก้ปวด ก็มากมายแล้ว

2 ช่วยให้ประชาชนมีสุขภาพที่ดีรื่นเมื่อคนเงี่ยงการกินยารักษาโรค จนเกิดโรครร่างเคียงต่าง ๆ
ประชาชนจะสุขสบาย

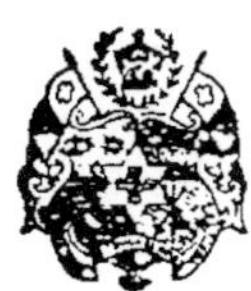

MINISTRY OF HEALTH, NUKU'ALOFA, TONGA.
(POTUNGAUE 'O E MO'UI)

P. O. Box 59
Nuku'alofa, Tonga.
Phone : 23-200
Fax : 24-291
Cable : MINHEALTH

Our Ref:

21st January, 1994

Dr. Laiyin Yan
California Medical Research Institute
1211 N. Vermont Ave. #207
Los Angeles
CA 90029

Dear Sir,

For the last 2½ years, I have used XH-1 to treat illnesses and achieved very good results.

The King of Tonga, liked this XH-1 therapeutic machine very much. His Majesty stated that this XH-1 therapeutic machine is very convienient to use, very safe, and very effective. His Majesty appreciated very much that California Medical Research Institute has donated 12 XH-1 therapeutic machines to be distributed to the Ministry of Health of Tonga, Tuvalu, and Nauru, and also very grateful that the government of the Republic of China and the California Medical Research Institute of the U.S. invited Dr. Laiyin Yan to come to teach the physicians on how to use the XH-1 therapeutic machine to treat-illnesses.

His Majesty hopes that, beginning of next year, more XH-1 therapeutic machines can be donated to the Ministry of Health of Tonga, Tuvalu, and Nauru, and have Dr. Laiyin Yan invited to teach the physicians of the Ministry of Health of the 3 nations.

Thank you

Sincerely

Dr. S. T. Puloka
Director of Health &
Royal Physician

Ministry of Health
Kingdom of Tonga

cc: Embassador of
    Republic of China

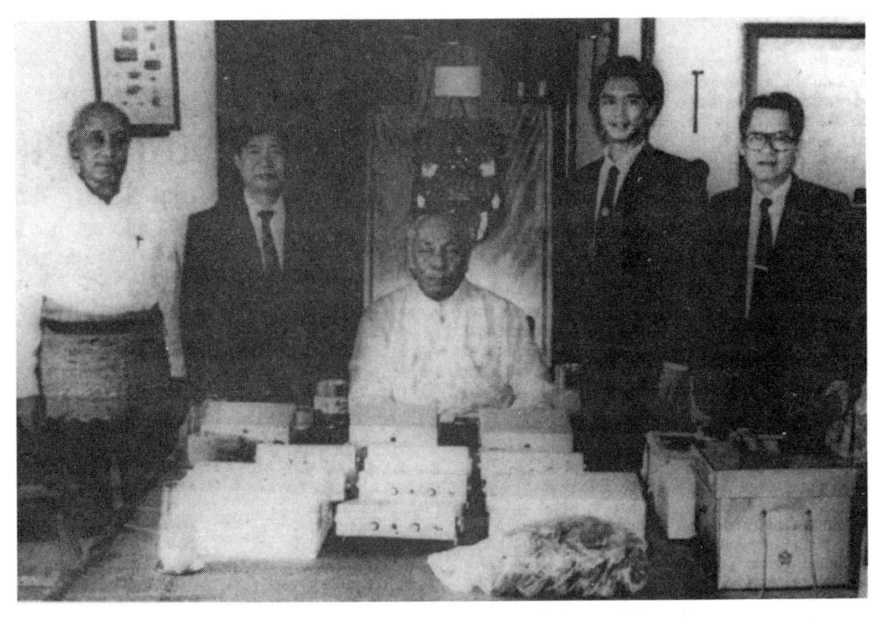

Prof. NGUYEN VIET
Director
National Institute
of Mental Health
Bach Mai Hospital
HANOI

Chairman
Psychiatry Department
HANOI Medical College

President
National Association
of Psychiatry,
Neurology and
Neurosurgery .

TELEPHONE :
Office No:62087
Home No:21079
Hanoi Viet Nam

Hanoi, January 29th ~~199~~ 1994

Mister SUI CHI LIN
Representative
TAIPEI Economic and Cultural Office
in Ha Noi SRV

Mister The Representative,

First of all, I would like to express our thanks for your precious assistance in inviting Doctor and Mrs LAIYIN YAN to visit our country and give us five XH-1 therapeutic machines.

After the therapeutic demonstration of Professor YAN in Ha Noi, we have witnessed the first good results of this machine.. We hope we will be able to apply it succesfully in the treatment of Drug Addicts, one of the most important therapeutic problems in our country.

At present there are many centres of Drug Addiction Treatment in Viet Nam.. We would like to demand once more your assistance for obtaining from California Medical Research Institute five more XH-1 machines for some of these centres.

With best regards

Yours sincerely,

Pr. NGUYEN VIET
President
National Association
of Psychiatry
Neurology and
Neurosurgery

Ha Noi SR Viet Nam

To: president of the Medical Research Institute of California

The favorable consideration by the Medical Research Institute of California, USA will be highly appreciated.

Sincerely,

Sui Chi Lin
Representative,
Taipei Economic & Cultural office
Hanoi, Vietnam

(TRANSLATED BY PETER SHIEH FROM CHINESE WORLD NEWS DAILY DATED DECEMBER 21, 1990)

SECRETARY-GENERAL TO THE PRESIDENT
OF THE REPUBLIC OF CHINA--
MR. YIEN-SHI TSIANG.
GRANTED AN AUDIENCE TO
ZHANG ZHENGMING AND YAN LAIYIN
TO PROBE FOR THE SOLUTION OF
AMPHETAMINE PROBLEM
AND GAVE ATTENTION TO DR. YAN'S
MEDICATION-FREE
DRUG ADDICTION THERAPY

The Honorable Captain and the drug treating expert, Zhang Zhengming and Dr. Yan Laiyin, respectively, of Thai representative group for the 3rd Joint Conference of the World Congress of Chinese Medicine and Pharmacy and the International Symposium on Acupuncture and Moxibustion have already returned to Bangkok.

While having a medical investigational tour in Kaohsiong, Secretary-General to the President-- Yien-shi Tsiang, arrived on December 5th to receive Zhang Zhengming and Yan Laiyin at the V.I.P. room. Due to Yan Laiyin's high medical skill in treating drug addiction without the use of medication, Secretary Yien-shi Tsiang gave attention to it.

During the reception, Secretary Yien-shi Tsiang showed great care about the "amphetamine flooding" problem in Taiwan. He discussed with Dr. Yan Laiyin about the solution to the problem. Dr. Yan and Zhang Zhengming showed great concern about Taiwan's drug problem, and spent one hour discussing about it.

After the reception, Secretary-General-- Mr. Yien-shi Tsiang invited Zhang Zhengming and Yan Laiyin to stay and take an information-exchange tour at Yuanshang Clinic and other areas. During the tour, with only one treatment, Dr. Yan's superior medical skill and the self-invented XH-1 qigong signal therapeutic machine were able to cure or relieve the strange and difficult to treat diseases, which were treated by other doctors with no good results, and achieve conspicuous results. All the medical experts and professors around were stunned, and felt that this is incredible.

Honorable Group Captain Zhang Zhengming and Dr. Yan already arrived back in Thailand by now. In the mean time, Dr. Yan is busy working on the thesis "The Clinical Application of Qigong Signal" for entering the 1991 International Qigong Conference. At the same time, he is discussing with the related departments and staffs about the problems and solutions of "amphetamine flooding".

According to the source, Zhang Zhengming and Yan Laiyin will visit Taiwan in the middle of next month. Besides attending the meeting, they will also academically answer questions from Secretary Yien-shi Tsiang.

40

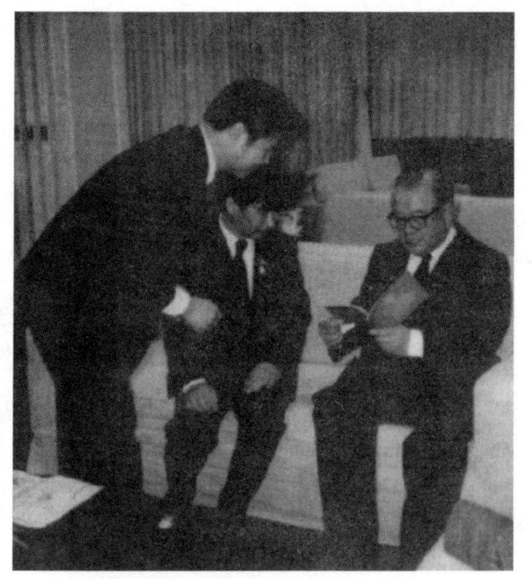

At the airport V.I.P. room, Secretary-General to the president of the republic of China, Mr. Yien-shi Tsiang (sitting to the right), receives specialized physician of the Republic of China, Dr. Laiyan Yan (sitting in the center), for more than an hour and gives attention to the Dr. Laiyin-invented medication-free XH-1 illness and drug-addiction therapy.

圖：總統府秘書長蔣彥士（右）十二月五日，在高雄機場接見張政銘和宴萊蔭醫師。

總統府秘書長蔣彥士
接見張政銘與宴萊蔭

探討安非他命問題解決之道
重視宴醫師無藥戒毒醫療法

【本報訊】泰國出席第三屆世界中國醫藥學會國際針灸研究會的名譽團長張政銘，戒毒專家宴萊蔭醫學博士，已於日前返回曼谷。

他們出席大會後在高雄醫療考察時，國府總統府秘書長蔣彥士，十二月五日特趕來高雄，在飛機場貴賓室接見了張政銘和宴萊蔭，由於宴醫師無藥戒毒的高深醫術，受到蔣彥士秘書長的關注。

接見時蔣秘書長對台灣現時「安非他命」泛濫的問題，深表關切，他與宴萊蔭醫師商討了有關解決問題的方法。宴醫師和張政銘名譽團長對台灣毒品泛濫問題表示非常憂視，整個會談達一小時之久。接見後蔣秘書長，特地請張團長和宴醫師留下來，安排到圓山診所和各地區參觀交流，在交流期間

，宴醫師高超的醫術，和他所發明的氣功信息治療儀，竟使一些久治不癒的疑難雜症，僅一次治療就痊癒，或使其症狀減輕，取得了明顯的療效，使在場的醫學專家和教授，驚奇萬分，感到不可思議。

名譽團長張政銘和宴萊蔭醫師現已回泰國。宴醫師，目前正在忙著寫醫學論文「氣功信息」，在臨床上的應用」，為參加八十年代全世界氣功大會作準備。同時正與有關部門和人員，研討「安·非他命」泛濫的問題和解決的方法。

據悉，張政銘和宴醫師，下月中旬將再次訪問台灣，除出會議之外，還將就蔣彥士秘書長提出的一些問題，提出學理上的回答。

SIAM TRANSLATION

สยาม ทรานสเลชั่น

57/4 Wireless Road (Opposite Ayuthaya Bank) Bangkok   10330

57/4 ถนนวิทยุ (ตรงข้ามธนาคารกรุงศรีฯ) เพลินจิต กรุงเทพฯ 10330

Tel. 2545582, 2501656

(Translation)

Translated from "Daily News" dated 10 April 1991, page 26.

<u>CURING DRUG ADDICTS WITH ELECTRICITY</u>

Bangkok Municipality succeeded in curing addicts with electricity.

Doctor Khajit Choopanya, Deputy Director of Health Department disclosed that Health Department had been trying to cure drug addicts by using low amperage electricity at the Drug Clinic of Public Health Center No. 19, Wongswwang 4 years ago with assistance from Dr. Yan Laiyin from Taiwan. There were about 100 heroin addicts joined the trial. Almost all of them were men.

Doctor Khajit said further that curing by using electric wire connected with low amperage machine, XH-1, with metal button at the end of the wire to stimulate body's cell to have reaction to the feeling will reduce symptom of drug addicts. He sees that this way of curing is good. Previously patients were cured by using methadone which is believe it is one kind of drug. Using electricity will not create any side effect to patients and major of them get better gradually. He will report to the administration and request them to increase this service, free of charge as usual, in other Public Health Centers. He added that Bangkok Municipality is the first in trying to cure addicts this way.

เดลินิวส์

รักษาพวกติดผงด้วยไฟฟ้า

ตระเวนตรวจ

ชุมชนวัดบรมนิวาส
ไม่มีปัญหาใดๆ

จราจรลัดจลาจล

จลาจลถนนเกษมราษฎร์

ถนนเกษมราษฎร์ เป็นถนนสายสั้น ๆ จากหน้าการท่าเรือแห่งประเทศไทยผ่านกรมการขุดภาคเรือมาถนนพระรามที่ ๔ ยาวไม่เกิน ๑ กม.

ไฟเหลือง

SIAM TRANSLATION

สยาม ทรานสเลชั่น

57/4 Wireless Road (Opposite Ayuthaya Bank) Bangkok   10330

57/4 ถนนวิทยุ (ตรงข้ามธนาคารกรุงศรีฯ) เพลินจิต กรุงเทพฯ 10330

Tel. 2515582, 2501656

(Translation)

Translated from "Daily News" dated 13 April 1991, page 22.

RESULT OF WORK ... NEW ERA OF BANGKOK MUNICIPALITY

<u>CURING DRUG ADDICTS WITH ELECTRICITY</u>

We have found that 90% of drug addicts are addicted to heroin which is considered the most dangerous kind of drug. Heroin are harmful to body and its process of taking can create complication easily. Government sections concerned and private sectors are fighting for decreasing the number of drug addicts. There are many ways of treating heroin addicts, by taking medicine, performing acupuncture, using herb to counteract the poison, but these ways sometimes create problems. Patients, in substitution for heroin, are addicted to the medicine used in their treatment.

At present, there is a new way of curing drug addicts that is by using electricity. Taiwanese doctor, Dr. Yan Laiyin, who introduced this method had brought the XH-1 machine and tried with patients at Drug Clinic of Public Health Center No. 19, Wong Sawang, which belongs to Bangkok Municipality. His machine looks like electrical adaptor, contained with low voltage electricity, designed by himself. At the adapter, there is one pole of electric wire divided into two metal ends. The end of the wire is made of metal using for electrifying various points of body. All together there are 16 machines and he had been trying for 4 years already.

Khun Suneephorn Anuttarakulvanich, Head of Social Worker at Drug Clinic, Public Health Center No. 19 said that normally clinic open at 8:00 a.m. but people come earlier than that. So she has to start treating before time because most of patients come with symptom of drug-in-need so badly. There are two types of patients, those who used to come and the new comers. Usually they have never asked anything. she will teach them how and where to electrify. The points are at cervical bone and at near the wrists. If patient had pain at which part she will electrify that place as well. After patients had learned from her they could do it themselves. Each patient will take about 5 minutes for electrifying. After that the symptom of drug-in-need will be over. Khun Suneephorn added that in each day there are about 100 patients, both men and women.   there are both teenagers and middle agers coming for treatment until the time of closing clinic at 11;30 a.m.

44

SIAM TRANSLATION

สยาม ทรานสเลชั่น

57/4 Wireless Road (Opposite Ayuthaya Bank) Bangkok   10330

57/4 ถนนวิทยุ (ตรงข้ามธนาคารกรุงศรีฯ) เพลินจิต กรุงเทพฯ 10330

Tel. 2545582, 2501656

(Translation)

My observation of the patients cured by electrifying, first person is a man of 26 years lived at Soi Saithong, Nonthaburi, addicted to drug since the last 3 years and he wanted to get out of it. He had been treated by medicine for 8 months. Last 3 days he changed to electrifying. When he first came to clinic, his face was pale, his hands and his voice were shaky. After electrifying for a while, we could understand his words better. He said he was all right, after that he rushed home. Second one was a women of 27 years old lived in Soi Kingpet, Phyathai. She came with one girl who has the same symptom. When she came she did not say anything, only pulled out the electric wire and electrified herself skillfully. After a while she started talking. She said she is a house wife. She wants to give up drug because when she was in need of drug, it was torturing. She would like to have this machine at home to treat her pain often so that she could recover soon. She said it reduced her pain like taking medicine. Third one is young man of 21 years old, living at Nonthaburi. He came by recommendation of his friend. He was addicted to drug for two years. He wanted to give up because he wanted to work. If he took drug he could not work, drug's reaction made him had no strength. When he came he said he was shivered by hot and cold feeling. He has got stomach ache, feeling like vomiting. The officer taught him how to electrify. After that five minutes he said he was all right. He said this way is easy and he will come back again. Another person lived in Soi Yim Prayoon, previously lived in Klong Toei. His occupation is vender. He said he thinks he is completely cured and he does not want to take drug any more. When he first came for electrifying he still took medicine. Later he had been treated by electrifying only. He said electrifying can cure his symptoms like medicine.

Doctor Kajit Chooopanya. Deputy Director of Health Department gave an opinion for using electrifying to cure heroin addicts that the result of 4 years trial is very satisfied. He said the reason to look for new way of treatment is because before Drug Clinics at various Public Health Centers used methadone in treating and they were afraid of its side effect since somebody said methadone is also another kind of drug. They had tried to investigate new way of treatment and had chance to try this way with assistance of Taiwanese Doctor, Yan Laiyin. The quality of this XH-1 machine is that it can detoxify, get rid of withdrawal, and curing complication which may be caused by various kind of pain. Patient who comes regularly will be absolutely cured, drug in their blood will be got rid of. This treatment is no harm and it is new

SIAM TRANSLATION

สยาม ทรานสเลชั่น

57/4 Wireless Road (Opposite Ayuthaya Bank) Bangkok 10330

57/4 ถนนวิทยุ (ตรงข้ามธนาคารกรุงศรีฯ) เพลินจิต กรุงเทพฯ 10330

Tel. 2545582, 2501656

(Translation)

treatment for Thailand. We can not increase our service due to budget shortage. We are planning to discuss about this matter with the administration concerned for financial support.

I Hope Government will realize the importance of helping drug addicts to get out of their hell and becoming strong and healthy citizen of the country in the future.

Donreudee Wongkiam
Reporter

ผลงาน...กทม.ยุคใหม่

รักษาขี้ยาด้วยไฟฟ้า...

ในจำนวนผู้ติดยาเสพติดทั้งหมด พบว่า ๙๐ เปอร์เซ็นต์คือผู้ที่เสพเฮโรอีน ซึ่งถือเป็นยาเสพติดที่มีพิษภัยต่อร่างกายรุนแรงที่สุด ทั้งโทษและกระบวนการเสพย่อมให้เกิดโรคแทรกซ้อนได้ง่าย เป็นปัญหาที่หน่วยงานทั้งภาครัฐและเอกชนพยายามรณรงค์เพื่อลดละเลิกยาเสพติดคอยู่ การรักษาผู้ติดยาเสพติดเฮโรอีนก็มีหลายวิธีด้วยกัน ทั้งกินยา ฝังเข็ม ถอนพิษด้วยสมุนไพร แต่การรักษาด้วยวิธีทางต่าง ๆ เหล่านั้น อาจเกิดปัญหาผู้เสพติดยาที่ใช้รักษาแทน

ขณะนี้มีการรักษาผู้ติดยาเสพติดด้วยวิธีใหม่คือการรักษาด้วยกระแสไฟฟ้า โดยการคิดค้นของ ดร.เยน โฮยัน เป็นวิเพทย์วิศวะชาวไต้หวัน ได้นำเครื่องมือมาทดลองรักษาให้ผู้ติดยาที่คลินิกยาเสพติดศูนย์บริการสาธารณสุข 17 วงศ์สว่าง

เป็นศูนย์บริการสาธารณสุขของ กท. เครื่องที่ใช้มีลักษณะคล้ายหม้อแปลงไฟฟ้าที่คิดค้นขึ้นเอง มีประจุไฟฟ้าอ่อนมากที่เครื่องจะมีที่เสียบ 1 สาย แยกเป็นขั้วบากขั้วลบ ที่ปลายสายไฟจะเป็นโลหะเพื่อใช้ขี้กับจุดต่าง ๆ มีทั้งหมด 16 เครื่อง ได้ทดลองรักษาผู้ป่วยมาเป็นเวลา 4 ปีแล้ว

คุณสุพักตร์ อนุตรกุลนิธิ หัวหน้านักสังคมสงเคราะห์ คลินิกยาเสพติดศูนย์ฯ 17 เล่าให้ฟังว่าศูนย์เปิดบริการเวลา 08.00 น. แต่จะมีผู้ติดยามารอเข้าคิวตั้งแต่เช้า คนที่มารับรักษาก่อนเวลาเพราะผู้ที่มานั้นจะเกิดอาการ "เสี่ยน" หรือต้องการเสพยาทุกคน ในแต่ละวันทั้งผู้หญิงมาแล้วและพิ่งมาครั้งแรกส่วนใหญ่จะไม่ค่อยสอบถามรายละเอียดอะไร จะให้คนสอนวิธีการขี้ให้ จุดที่ใช้ก็คือที่ท้ายทอย และที่ข้อมือ หากผู้ป่วยปวดกระตุกปวดร้าวใหม่มาก หรือปวดท้องก็จะใช้ขึ้นร่วมดังกล่าวด้วยเมื่อรู้วิธีแล้วครั้งต่อไปขนมปลือกจะสำเร็จแรง คนหนึ่งจะใช้เวลาที่ประมาณ 5 นาที หลังจากนั่นเมื่ออาการเสี่ยนยาของเขาจะหาย

อาการปวดได้เหมือนกับกินยาที่ตนเคยมารักษาที่คลินิกยาเสพติดต่าง ๆ เด็กหนุ่มอีกคนหนึ่ง อายุ 21 ปี อยู่นนทบุรี มารักษาครั้งแรกบอกเพื่อนแนะนำให้มา ติดยามา 2 ปี แล้วอยากจะเลิกเพราะอยากทำงานที่ผ่านมาเสพแล้วทำงานไม่ได้ ไม่มีแรง หงึ่ยเยากด้วน ขณะที่มาบอก รู้สึกร้อน ๆ หนาว ๆ ตลื่นไส้ ปวดท้องฯ หลังจากที่เจ้าหน้าที่แนะนำการขี้ให้ประมาณ 8 นาทีอาการของเขาก็ดีขึ้น เมื่อถูกถามกับบอกหายแล้ว บอกความรู้สึกที่รักษาด้วยไฟฟ้าน่ำง่ายดี แล้วจะมาอีก ยังรายบ้านอยู่ในซอยยิ้มประยูร นนทบุรี เดิมอยู่กองขลดอาชีพทำขาย กล่าวว่าขณะนี้คนคิดว่า

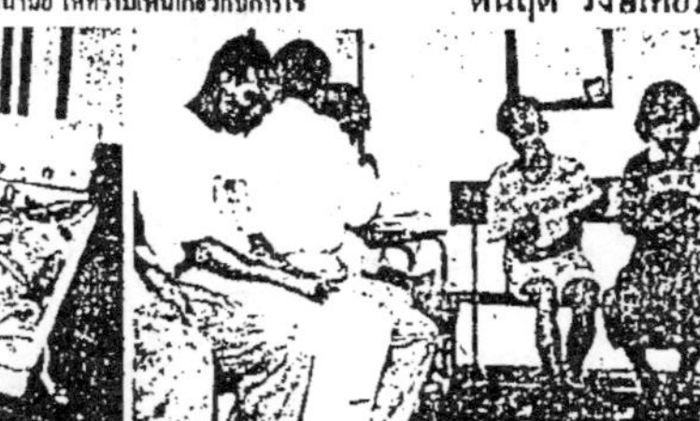

ตัวเองหายขาดแล้ว ไม่นึกอยากเสพยาอีก มารักษาด้วยไฟฟ้าก็แค่เริ่มทดลองช่วงแรกใช้ควบไปกับกินยา เพราะระยะหลัง ๆ อาการอยากน้อยลงกี่ใช้ไฟฟ้าเชื่ออย่างเดียวการใช้ไฟฟ้าทำให้หายอาการได้เช่นกัน

ด้าน นพ.ขจิต ชุปัญญา รอง ผอ.- สำนักอนามัย ให้ความเห็นเกี่ยวกับการใช้ไฟฟ้ารักษาผู้ติดยาว่ายิ่งอ้นว่า จากที่ได้ทดลองมา 4 ปี ผลที่ได้เป็นที่น่าพอใจ ปัจจุบันกลืนนักต่าง ๆ ตามศูนย์บริการสาธารณสุขที่ให้การรักษาอยู่จะรักษาด้วยยาเมทาโดนซึ่งเป็นยาทดแทนเฮโรอีนก็เกรงว่าจะเกิดผลข้างเคียง ติดยาตามมา จึงได้คิดหาวิธีใหม่ ๆ จึงมีการทดลองวิธีดังกล่าว โดยความ-ช่วยเหลือจากหมอไต้หวัน คุณสมบัติของเครื่องดังกล่าวสามารถถอนพิษยา ขจัดอาการและรักษาโรคแทรกซ้อน อันเกิดจากความเจ็บปวดต่าง ๆ ผู้มารักษาประจำพิษยาในร่างกายก็จะหมดไป อีกว่าเป็นวิธีที่ไม่ก่อให้เกิดอันตรายใด ๆ และเป็นการรักษาวิธีใหม่ในประเทศไทยที่ยังไม่ขยายบริการขณะนี้เพราะติดขัดเรื่องงบประมาณเครียมหารือกับผู้บริหารให้รัฐบาลสนับสนุน

หวังว่ารัฐบาลคงจะเห็นความสำคัญช่วยผู้ติดยาให้รอดพ้นจากขุมนรกระที่เพื่อกลับมาเป็นพลเมืองดีของชาติต่อไป

ดนฤดี วงษ์เกี่ยม

(TRANSLATED FROM TAIWAN SHING SHENG NEWS DATED DECEMBER 17, 1990)

NARCOTIC FLOODING
FOR SEVERAL YEARS, THE THAI GOVERNMENT
HAS BEEN WORKING HARD TO HANDLE IT
BY USING THE QIGONG SIGNAL THERAPEUTIC MACHINE
WITH MEDICATION-FREE METHOD OF TREATMENT FOR
DISEASES AND DRUG ADDICTION,
THE EFFICACY RATE REACHED 90%

--------------By Chang Hai-Sheng

(Translated by Peter Shieh)
Taiwan Shing Sheng News Staff

Recently amphetamine is flooding on the campus of Taiwan. Because Thailand, which is located in South East Asia next to the narcotic producing Golden Triangle, also has the problem of having their citizens taking heroine and other narcotics. In the recent 4 years, the Thai government has been using the qigong signal therapeutic machine with medication-free qigong method of treatment for diseases and drug addiction, and had good treatment results.

According to Dr. Yan Laiyin, a doctor of Chinese medicine from Thailand, he inspected the therapy used in the Narcotic clinics provided by the United Nation and found out that it does not have good results and has adverse effects. He then tried acupuncture, electrical acupuncture machine, and qigong signal machine to treat illnesses and drug addiction. Finally, he invented his own XH-1 signal therapeutic machine with medication-free qigong method of treatment for diseases and drug addiction.

Since november 2, 1986, Thailand has been using this therapy for 4 whole years, and treated over 50,000 cases, include the regular patients that are not drug addicts. According to the statistic from the Bangkok Metropolitan Department of Health, Thailand, the efficacy rate reached over 90%, All the clinical statistic data were saved into the Bangkok Metropolitan Government's computer file.

In 1985, this doctor of Chinese medicine risked his life entering the Golden Triangle of Burma all by him self to study the withdrawal syndrome and the ways to treat it. He pointed out that the important point of treating drug addiction is to relieve the addicts' illnesses first (whether the illness is drug induced or non-drug induced) in to achieve the goal of treating illnesses and drug addiction; and then further rehabilitate their health so they can live and work like normal people. As far as what the principle of this disease and drug treating therapy is, we apply the specific signal to the related locations of the human body to drive the various physiological functions back to normal. From the elimination of the 17 illnesses of drug withdrawal syndrome to avoid mortality due to internal organ spasm, which causes hemorrhage and the heart failure, at the same time, it relieves other illnesses and achieved the goal of treating illnesses and drug addiction.

According Qigong Master Yan, who modestly claimed to be an adviser of the United Headquarter of Chinese qigong of Thailand, this therapy has the following characteristics:

1. Within a short period of 5 to 15 minutes, it can relieve the illnesses of the drug withdrawal syndrome and eliminate the severe life-threatening conditions of the severe drug withdrawal syndrome, and effectively rescued several drug quitters' life. There has never been any mortality for all 4 years.

2. Within 4 to 7 days, it can completely eliminate the 17 illnesses of drug withdrawal syndrome, and relieve various types of other illnesses (whether the illnesses are drug induced or non drug induced).

3. After the treatment for drug addiction, follow by 7 more days of rehabilitation treatment, almost all the drug quitters have improved food appetite, sleep, spirited feel after awakening, physical strength, sexual function, feel comfortable, and able to live and work like normal people.

4. It is quick and effective for conditioning the physiological functions, driving them normal, and relieving the symptoms. Clinically, besides for treating drugs, it can also be used for emergency rescue, treating illnesses, and rehabilitation.

5. The biggest characteristic is that the more obvious the symptom is, the more conspicuous the result of this therapy has.

6. By treating illnesses and drug addiction and emergency rescue without using medication, a lot of medication and cost can be saved.

7. It is easy to use, the patients can operate themselves.

8. It has no danger, because it has the right amount of amperage.

(NOTE: The writer followed the members of the 3rd Conference of the International Acupuncture of Chinese Medical Association and toured at the Chinese herbal structure.   At the Ching Jing Farm Citizen's Hotel, the writer actually saw Dr. Yan using this XH-1 therapeutic machine to treated a female college student's sprained ankle and foot due to mountain climbing. She needed the help of other people to lift her and could still walk with only one leg. After one half hour treatment, she could walk nearly perfectly normally by her self. That night, Dr. Yan also gave the farmers and their relatives free treatment.)

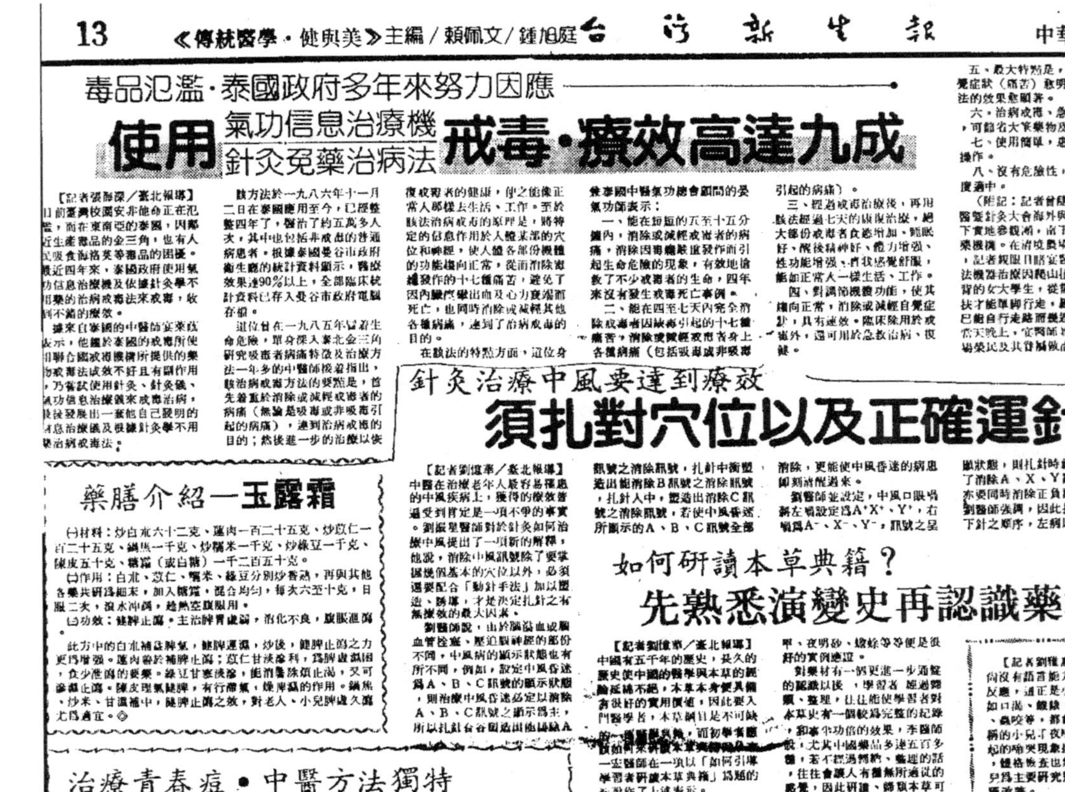

毒品氾濫‧泰國政府多年來努力因應

使用氣功信息治療機　針灸免藥治病法　戒毒‧療效高達九成

【記者張麗深／臺北報導】目前臺灣校園安非他命正在氾濫，而在東南亞的泰國，因鄰近生產毒品的金三角，也有人以吸食海洛英等毒品的困擾。最近四年來，泰國政府使用氣功信息治療機及依據針灸學不用藥的治病戒毒法來戒毒，收到不錯的療效。

據來自泰國的中醫師表示，他鑑於泰國的戒毒所使用聯合國或福慧機構所提供的藥物戒毒法成效不好且有副作用，乃嘗試使用針灸、針灸儀、氣功信息治療機來戒毒治病，最後發展出一套他自己發明的信息治療儀及根據針灸學不用藥治病戒毒法。

該方法於一九八六年十一月二日在泰國應用至今，已經整整四年了，醫治了約五萬多人次，其中也包括非戒毒的普通病患者。根據泰國曼谷市政府衛生廳的統計資料顯示，醫療效果達90%以上，全部臨床統計資料已存入曼谷市政府電腦存檔。

這位曾在一九八五年冒著生命危險，單身深入泰北金三角研究吸毒者病痛特徵及治療方法一年多的中醫師後指出，戒治病戒毒方法的要點是，首先着重於消除或減輕戒毒者的病痛（無論是吸毒或非吸毒引起的病痛），達到治病戒毒的目的；然後進一步的治療以恢復吸毒者的健康，使之能像正常人那樣去生活、工作。至於信息法治病戒毒的原理是，將特定的信息作用於人體某部的穴位和神經，使人體各部份機體的功能趨向正常，從而消除毒癮發作的十七種痛苦，避免了因內臟突變出血及心力衰竭而死亡，也同時消除或減輕其他各種病痛，達到了治病戒毒的目的。

在信息法的特點方面，這位身兼泰國中醫氣功總會顧問的吳氣功師表示：

一、能在短短的五至十五分鐘內，消除或減輕戒毒者的病痛，消除因毒癮驟區發作而引起生命危險的現象，有效地搶救了不少戒毒者的生命，四年來沒有發生戒毒死亡事例。

二、能在四至七天內完全消除戒毒者因缺毒引起的十七種痛苦，消除或減輕戒毒者身上各種病痛（包括吸毒或非吸毒引起的病痛）。

三、經過戒毒治療後，再用信息法經過七天的信息治療，絕大部份戒毒者食慾增加、睡眠好、醒後精神好、體力增強、性功能增強、有我感覺舒服，能如正常人一樣生活、工作。

四、對調節機體功能，使其趨向正常，消除或減輕自覺症狀，具有速效。臨床應用於戒毒外，還可用於急救治病、復健。

五、最大特點是，患者的自覺症狀（痛苦）愈明顯，信息療法的效果愈顯著。

六、治病戒毒，急救不用藥物，可節省大筆藥物及費用開支。

七、使用簡單，患者可自己操作。

八、沒有危險性，因電流強度適中。

（附記：記者曾隨第三屆中醫暨針灸大會海外與會人員南下實地參觀，南下參觀中醫藥機構。在消境藥場國民賓館，記者親眼目睹宴醫師用其信息機器治療因跌出扭傷腳踝而背的女大學生，從需要勞人攙扶才能單腳行走，歷半小時後已能自行走路而幾近無痠麻。當天晚上，宴醫師慈免費為農場榮民及其眷屬做治療。）

針灸治療中風要達到療效

須扎對穴位以及正確運針

【記者劉懷華／臺北報導】中醫在治療老年人最容易罹患的中風疾病上，獲得的療效普遍受到肯定是一項不爭的事實。劉振星醫師對於針灸如何治療中風提出了一項新的解釋，他說，消除中風訊號除了要掌握這幾個基本的穴位以外，必須還要配合「動針手法」加以塑造、誘導，才是決定扎針之有無療效的最大因素。

劉醫師說，由於腦溢血或血管栓塞、壓迫腦神經的部份不同，中風病的顯示狀態也有所不同，例如，設定中風昏迷為A、B、C訊號的顯示狀態，則治療中風昏迷必定以消除A、B、C訊號之顯示為主，所以扎針合谷圍造出消除A訊號之消除訊號，扎針中衝塑造出能消除B訊號之消除訊號，扎針人中，塑造出消除C訊號之消除訊號，若使中風昏迷所顯示的A、B、C訊號全部消除，更能使中風昏迷的病患即刻消醒過來。

劉醫師並設定，中風口眼喎斜左頰設定為A⁺X⁺、Y⁺，右頰為A⁻、X⁻、Y⁻，訊號之呈現狀態，則扎針時就要配合除了消除A、X、Y訊號之外，亦要同時消除正負訊號，劉醫師強調，因此扎針時要守下針之順序，左頰以右側為主。

如何研讀本草典籍？

先熟悉演變史再認識藥材

【記者劉雅惠／臺北報導】中國有五千年的歷史，長久的歷史使中國的醫學與本草的經驗延續不絕。本草本身便具備有很好的實用價值，因此要入門醫學者，本草綱目是不可缺。而初學者要如何來研讀本草典籍呢？一位醫師在一項以「如何引導學習者研讀本草典籍」為題的演說作了上述表示。

對藥材有一個更進一步通盤的認識以後，學習者越過細難、整理，讓他從學醫者對本草史有一個較為完整的記錄，和事半功倍的效果，李醫師說，尤其中國藥品多達五百多種，若不經過辨解、整理的話，往往會讓人有繁無所適從的感覺，因此研讀、歸類本草可甲、夜明砂、蟋蟀等等便是很好的實例遊應。

藥膳介紹—玉露霜

㈠材料：炒白朮六十二克、蓮肉一百二十五克、炒苡仁一百二十五克、鍋焦一千克、炒糯米一千克、炒綠豆一千克、陳皮五十克、糖霜（或白糖）一千二百五十克。

㈡作用：白朮、苡仁、糯米、綠豆分別炒香熟，再與其他各藥共研得細末，加入糖霜，混合均勻，每次六至十克，日服二次，放水沖調，趁熱空腹服用。

㈢功效：健脾止瀉。主治脾胃虛弱，消化不良，腹脹泄瀉。

此方中的白朮補益脾氣，健脾運濕，炒後，健脾止瀉之力更爲增強。蓮肉善於補脾止瀉；苡仁甘淡滲利，爲脾虛濕困、食少便溏的要藥。綠豆甘寒淸熱，能消暑除煩止渴，又可滲濕止瀉。陳皮理氣健脾，有行帶氣，燥脾濕的作用。鍋焦、炒米、甘溫補中，健脾止瀉之效，對老人、小兒脾虛久瀉尤爲適宜。◇

治療青春痘‧中醫方法獨特

TO WHOM IT MAY CONCERN:

A NEW LIFE IS BEGINNING FOR ME AFTER USING THE XH-1
REHABILITATION MACHINE.
I, Virginia B. Ensor, have been using the XH-1 Rehabilitation
machine for about two months and would like to let everyone
know of the wonderfull relief I am getting and improvement in my
condition.

I have had a heart condition for more than 30 years, becomIng
more severe in the past year. Most recently I went through a
traumatic family emotional experience resulting in a move from
the home to a hotel. Much anger and heated discussions
culminated in an extremely nervous and tense condition where I
virtually lost control of my emotions. After a day or so I
experienced severe dizzyness with the slightest movement of my
head or when sitting up. Even while lying in bed I had a vivid
feeling of falling and sometimes everthing would go black. I
called Dr. Yan for this emergency situation. The dizzyness
actually started about 5 days before as the tension was
building up; but with about an hour of treatment with the XH-1
machine I could stand normally. Most all of the dizzyness was
gone and I had regained control. Dr. Yan recommended that
treatment continue for about ten days and it is expected that
the problems will remain in control for an extended period.

My introduction to the XH-1 machine:
Almost 40 years ago I was the driver of a car involved in a
near fatal accident. The car was totally destroyed and I was
nearly killed. The injury list included broken ribs, collapsed
lung, skull fracture, ruptured bladder, ruptured diaphragm,
fractured pelvic, many contusions and bruises over the body. I
was in a coma for 5 days and received last rights of the
catholic church.

Over the years these injuries and the normal flow of living led
to such maladies as internal intestinal and stomach disorders,
hysterectomy, cancer with a radical mastectomy, 3 times
fractured knee and leg (reported to be partially caused by early
osteoporosis from chemo therapy), and arthritis with
degenerative spine.

In recent months of this year the pain and discomfort
drastically increased to where I could not bear to walk. My
feet were hurting and burning as if on hot coals and pain
extending up through my legs, knees and back. Over the past
years the medical doctors have continued to prescribe pain
killers and muscle relaxers but could do little toward controlling
the continued degeneration of my condition. On a friend's
suggestion, I went to the acupuncture clinic at South Baylo
University in Garden Grove, CA.

Three acupuncture treatments were received at 5 day intervals.
When leaving the clinic after a treatment, I felt worse than when
I came and also through most of the next day.   That evening
my condition improved and lasted 2 more days before it started
to deterioate. By the fifth day I felt bad again but another
treatment was due. This cycle repeated for the 3 treatments.
Because my condition was not realy improved, on the day for the
fourth treatment I was referred by the supervising doctor to
Doctor Yan Laiyin, who is a Research Professor at the
University, and his assistant Peter Shieh. They were unwrapping
a machine, the XH-1 Rehabilitation machine, which had just been
shipped to the clinic. It was suggested that I try the machine
because of my serious problem of such long time origin.

Several machines were used simultaneously at several points
over my body that day. After about 2 hours of treatment, I got
up, by myself from the table and could walk without a cane or
aid. My back pain was virtually gone, at least the way that I
was used to feeling. It was recommended that I continue the
treatment for several days to evaluate the results.

With accupuncture I was totally exhausted after the treatment,
with the XH-1 machine it was the reverse; I am relaxed and
enthusiastic about life. The next day I was happy to return to
the clinic for the machine treatment. I drove by myself, which
was virtually a new experience for me since the past year or
so. On examination I found that I did still have some back pain,
but not nearly so severe and in different locations than
yesterday. Treatment proceeded again for about 2 hours at new
locations of pain and again I left feeling better than ever.

Doctor Yan told me that I should continue treatment for 32 days
since my condition resulted from the accident about 40 years
ago. During the next month or more I continued to improve and
gradually increased the time between treatments with the XH-1
machine.

While at the clinic I watched several patients come in for
treatment for back, arms, shoulders, legs and other pains. On
leaving the clinic after using the XH-1 machine, all of them spoke
of greatly improved conditions with easier and more extended
movement.

I BELIEVE THAT THIS XH-1 MACHINE HAS OPENED UP A NEW LIFE FOR
ME, I AM READY TO START LIVING AGAIN. Friends that see me now
don't immediately recognize me. They remember my previous
depressed look on my face and that I was barely able to walk
with a cane; I required a wheelchair when neccessary to go more
than a few feet.

Virginia B. Ensor
Virginia B. Ensor
1425 Springfield Apt A
Upland, CA 91786, U.S.A.

virginia.tes

ENEMY OF THE QUESTIONABLE
AND DIFFICULT TO TREAT DISEASES
--XH THERAPY

Dr. Yan Laiyin
Translated by Peter Shieh

NOTE: This thesis was requested by the King of Thailand and the
Secretary-General to the President of the Republic of China--
Mr. Yien-shi Tsiang.

THE STRANGE LEFT-AND-RIGHT TEMPERATURE DIFFERENCE OF A HUMAN
BODY

On June 15th, 1990, the Bangkok Metropolitan Department of
Health transferred a patient here. Swing Suwannanont, a 63 years
old male Thai citizen and an official of the United Nation,
complained that his left side of the body felt hot, and the right
side felt cold. When relaxed at night during sleep, the left
side became extremely hot, and the right side became extremely
cold, therefore, he was not being able to sleep. This agony was
so difficult to bear with that he had to live on sleeping pills
and narcotics. He has been to the U.S., Japan, England, and
China for treatment. It has been 3 years, but instead of getting
better, the illness only got worse, and he suffered a lot. The
transferred medical file stated: The temperature difference
between the left and right sides of the body is 4.3 degree
Celsius, there are no other abnormalities on the rest of the
body, include the cerebrum. I touched his limbs on both sides
with my hand and felt the obvious temperature difference between
his left and right side of the body. This is usually what people
called "a strange disease which its etiology cannot be detected".
By using the XH therapy, he was completely relieved and back to
normal in 32 days.

A PERSON THAT COLLAPSES RIGHT AFTER SITTING UP

On December 11th, 1990, Mr. Chian, a 75 years old male
patient of Taipei City, was hospitalized 2 years before and
diagnosed as having stoke due to cerebral embolism. He now
suffered from not being able to sit up after lying down, and
collapsing right after sitting up. In order to sit up
continuously, he would need someone else to hold him leaning on a
chair. After only one 1 hour of XH therapy, this symptom was
eliminated, and his health was back to normal.

A PERSON WHO LOST SENSATION ON THE RIGHT FOOT

On March 8th, 1991, Somchai Kornnimitr, a 27 years old male
patient who lost sensation on his right foot came to the clinic.
He has been treated in a hospital for over 3 months with no
improvement, and worse, the area with lost sensation was
expanding. Due to the lost of sensation, he fell often when
walking, and did not even know when his shoe slipped off his
foot. The hospital diagnosed him as sensory neuritis of the
right foot. After checking his condition thoroughly, we found
out that he could walk with his right foot but with completely

lost of pain sensation. After 2 XH therapies, this illness was
completely relieved.

THE STRANGE XH THERAPY
The diseases mentioned above could not be relieve by some
hospitals, but why can it be relieved by XH therapy? What was
going on here?
There is a famous saying from Chinese medicine, "If qi and
blood don't free flow, then pain appears." This is saying that
qi and blood inside the normal person travel continuously, and if
qi and blood free flow, then the person must be healthy. If qi
and blood do not flow freely, then illness/pain appears. In the
term "qi and blood", the word "blood" obviously is the blood and
the word "qi", according to the proofs from modern science,
stands for the traveling electrons inside the human body. (for
detailed information, please refer to the thesis "REVISITING
QIGONG SIGNAL AND ITS CLINICAL THERAPY").
If the electrical resistance, capacity, or conduction on
certain parts of the body had any abnormal change, which also
means the lack of free flow of the qi and blood was produced,
then the electric wave would deviate from normal, and clinically
various types of symptoms of illnesses would appear.
Therefore, throughout the history, people who have mastered
qigong use their mind power to move the qi, which is the electron
flow, to where the illnesses or pains are located, to free flow
the qi and blood, to drive the abnormal electromagnetic wave to
normal, and achieve the goal of rehabilitating to normal
mechanism of the body.
XH therapy is a kind of method of treatment which sends a
kind of qigong imitating electric wave accurately into the ill
location of the body to free flow the qi and blood, to
rehabilitate the body functions back to normal, and to relieve
the illnesses.
XH therapy has the characteristics of qigong therapy.

THE IMPORTANT POINT OF THE XH THERAPY
Because XH therapy rehabilitates the abnormal parts of the
body back to normal, the important point of the XH therapy is to
directly and accurately send the qigong imitating electric wave
into the ill or related locations of the body. Therefore, during
treatment, it is very important to let the patient point to the
painful or ill locations and describe about the illness in great
details. The more accurately the patient point to the ill spot,
the more thoroughly describing the illness, and the more
accurately the electrodes are placed, the more conspicuous the
treatment result will be. If the ill locations are not being
pointed to accurately, and not able to send the electric wave
accurately to the ill locations, then the treatment result would
be less effective, but with absolutely no danger. It is simply
to say that the important point of the XH therapy is similar to
that of qigong therapy. Treat wherever the illness is.

THE ATTACK OF "THE STRANGE LEFT-AND-RIGHT TEMPERATURE DIFFERENCE OF A HUMAN BODY"

From the Chinese medical point of view, a normal person's qi and blood flow on both sides of the body should be symmetrical. In this case, there was temperature difference between the left and right. It means there was a change in the electrical resistance, capacity, or conduction on one side of the body, creating imbalance of the qi and blood flow, and producing the temperature difference between the left and right sides of the body.

According to the pattern of "movement of the body produces heat", we are sure that the cold right hand side of the body was having lack of qi and blood circulation. So we applied the electric wave of XH therapy to the important meridian points and nerve locations of the right hand side of the body and limbs. Conspicuous result was produced after one therapy. After 32 therapies, all the symptoms were completely relieved. It has been a year and 2 months since the problem was eliminated, the patient is still very healthy. How would the western medicine treat this disease?

THE ATTACK OF "A PERSON THAT COLLAPSE RIGHT AFTER SITTING UP"

From the Chinese medical point of view, this case was mainly due to lack of qi and blood flow in the locations and motor nerves both of which controls the setting position. Therefore, as long as we can normalize the electrical resistance, capacity, and conduction of these parts of the body, we can eliminate the symptom.

Therefore, we sent the electric wave of XH therapy to the related locations. Only after one hour of treatment, the patient was rehabilitated to normal. The patient tried to lie down and sit up 3 times, and performed normally. It has been more than 10 months since this patient was completely relieved, he is still very healthy. How would the western medicine treat this disease?

THE ATTACK OF "A PERSON WHO LOST SENSATION ON THE RIGHT FOOT"

From the Chinese medical point of view, wherever there is illness, that is where the lack of free flow of qi and blood appears. As far as XH therapy is concerned, to device the methodology is, to say the least, simple. We applied the electric wave from the XH therapeutic machine through the large surface net electrode on the patient's right foot and leg. After the first treatment, the patient's basic sensory function of the right foot was already back to normal. After the second treatment, even the pain sensory function of the right foot was equal to that of the left foot, and the symptom was completely eliminated and back to normal. It has been 6 months since the symptom was eliminated. Today, the right foot is still normal. How would the western medicine treat this disease?

THE QI-BLOOD THEORY OF CHINESE MEDICINE IS WORTH GIVING ATTENTION TO

According to the analysis of the above medical cases, it proved that some diseases can neither be explained nor be treated by western medicine. However, they can be explained by the qi-blood theory of Chinese medicine. Starting with the qi-blood theory, by using the XH therapy, some diseases can be, indeed, treated very easily and relieved very quickly.

WHERE DID THE CERVICAL SPUR GO?

Of course some medical cases can be explained by the qi-blood theory, but not by today's science.

For the last 4 years or more, we have received 31 patients with cervical spur. This kind of patients have stiff neck, and are not able to turn the head left or right. If they needed to look at their side views, they would have to turn their whole body.

According to qi-blood theory, wherever there is illness, that location must have the lack of free flow of qi and blood. If the neck is stiff and cannot allow the head to turn, then obviously there is lack of free flow of qi and blood in the neck. Consequently, according to the important point of XH therapy, we should send the electric wave into the ill location--the neck. The result showed miracles. Almost all the patients had their symptoms relieved in 14 to 32 days. When the hospital retook the X-ray on the cervical, it show no spur. Then where did the spur go?

MIRACLES HAPPEN EVERYDAY

This type of miracles happen everyday at the 12th Narcotic Clinic of Bangkok. For the last 4 years or more, the total number of people who heard about its reputation, came to the clinic, and ask to be treated by the XH therapy on their illnesses or drug addiction has reached over 60,000. Especially people with either strange diseases which the etiology is unknown or certain types of strange and difficult to treat diseases, by using the XH therapy to treat them, the efficacy reached over 95%, and for drug addiction treatment, the efficacy is even higher at over 99%.

For treating the following 21 diseases, XH therapy has over 95% efficacy rate:

1. Certain heart diseases 2. high blood pressure 3. Low blood pressure 4. headache 5. migraine 6. dizziness 7. Menier's syndrome 8. glaucoma 9. insomnia 10. neck pain 11. stiff neck 12. allergic rhinitis 13. sprain 14. back pain 15. joint pain 16. arthredema 17. stomach disorders 18. nausea 19. dysmenorrhea 20. strange diseases which the etiology is unknown 21. psychological disorders due to meditation.

XH therapy has over 90% efficacy rate on relieving the 17 illnesses of the severe heroine withdrawal syndrome:
1. headache 2. dizziness 3. sleepiness 4. yawning
5. sneezing 6. neck pain 7. spine pain 8. lower back pain
9. muscle spasm of the limbs 10. abdominal pain 11. cramp of the internal organs 12. nausea 13. tight chest 14. chest pain
15. palpitation 16. cold sweat with coldness of the limbs 17. weakness.

WE DO NOT TAKE PATIENTS WITHOUT SEVERE ILLNESS
Due to the supply shortage of the XH therapeutic machine, we can only take 128 patients each day. In the mean time, we mainly take patients who want to quit drug use, because narcotic has too much effect the safety of the society.

According to the rule of the government, we can only, according to the condition of the illness, take a limited number of the other patients which hospitals could not diagnose the etiology, the condition of the illness is severe, and cannot be relieved by other therapies. In the mean time, the government is trying to solve this problem and expand the XH therapy to more clinics and hospitals. By that time, the area of Thailand must be able to satisfy more patients's request.

Dr. Yan Laiyin
Specialized Physician of Department of Health
Bangkok Metropolitan Administration, Thailand
October 1, 1991

Tel: (662)585-1672, 588-5068
Fax: (662)588-5068

疑難症的剋星——ＸＨ療法

ＤＲ．ＹＡＮ ＬＡＩＹＩＮ晏萊蔭博士
泰國曼谷市衛生廳專家醫師

奇異的人體左右溫差

一九九〇年六月十五日，曼谷市衛生廳批轉來一位病人，泰國籍的聯合國官員 SWING SUTANNANONT，６３歲，男，病人主訴身體左邊熱，右邊冷，晚上睡覺，靜下來，更覺左邊熱得厲害，右邊冷得厲害，無法入睡，其痛苦難以忍受，靠安眠藥、麻醉藥度日。曾去美國、日本、英國、中國大陸治療過，至今已二年多了，病非且沒有治好，病情反而越來越嚴重，精神很痛苦。轉診單上寫著：左右兩邊溫差達４.３℃，身體其他各部位，包括大腦，均未發現不正常情況。我用手摸一下，明顯地感到左右兩邊肢體一邊冷、一邊熱。這就是通常所稱的查無病因的怪病，經用ＸＨ療法醫治，３２天完全恢復正常。

坐起來就倒下的人

一九九〇年十二月十一日，在台北市，有一位病人錢××，７５歲，男，病人於二年多前病發住院，醫院診斷為中風，是腦血管阻塞造成，現在的症狀是，睡下就起不來，坐起來就倒下，必須有人幫助，扶他坐在靠背椅子上，才能坐穩，經用ＸＨ療法醫治，僅治療一小時，症狀就消除，恢復健康。

右腳失去知覺的人

一九九一年三月八日，門診來了一位病人SOMCHAI KORNNIMITR，２７歲，男，病人主訴右腳失去知覺，已在×××醫院治療了三個多月了，非但沒有好轉，失去知覺的範圍反而越來越擴大了，而且由於失去知覺，所以走路時經常容易跌倒，掉了鞋子也不知道，醫院診斷病人右腳感覺神經炎，我們詳細檢查了病情，發覺病人右膝能跨步走路，但對痛覺反應消失。經用ＸＨ療法醫治，僅治療二次就恢復健康了。

奇怪的ＸＨ療法

上述這些病，某些大醫院沒法治癒，為什麼用ＸＨ療法，竟能使病人恢復健康，這到底是怎麼一回事呢？

中醫有句名言，氣血不通則痛，此話的意思是說，正常人的氣血，在人體內不斷地在運動。氣血通，人必健，氣血不通，病痛發生。氣血的血，理所當然指的是血。這裡所指的氣，現代科學已證實就是人體內電子的運動。（詳見論文：再論氣功信息與臨床治療）

人體某部位的電阻、電容、電導值發生了不正常的變化，也就是產生了氣血不通的現象，其電波就異於正常，在臨床上就表現出各種病痛的症狀。

所以歷來之氣功修練者，就是用念力將氣，也就是電子流，運至病痛之部位，去疏通氣血，使不正常的電磁波集向正常，達到使機體恢復正常的目的。

ＸＨ療法，就是將一種模仿氣功的電波，準確地輸入到病痛部位，疏通氣血，使機體恢復正常，使病痛減輕或消除的一種治療方法。

ＸＨ療法，具有氣功古療法的特點。

ＸＨ療法的治療要點

因為ＸＨ療法是使不正常的機體部位恢復正常，所以ＸＨ療法的治療要點，就是將模仿氣功的電磁波，直接地，準確地輸入病痛部位，或有關的部位。所以在治療時，要求患者準確地指出病痛的部位和詳細敘述病情是十分重要的。病痛部位指得越準確，病痛敘述得越詳細，治療電極按放位置越準確，治療效果就越明顯。如病痛部位指得不準，使電波無法準確輸入病痛部位，治療效果就差一點，但絕對沒有危險性。簡單的說，ＸＨ療法的治療要點，如同用氣功治病的法則一樣，那裡有病痛，就治療那裡。

"奇異的人體左右溫差"之攻克

這個病例從中醫角度來看，正常人左右肢體之氣血流通，應是對稱平衡的，現在發生左右溫差，就是由於人體某一側某部位的電阻，電容，電導值發生變化，造成左右肢體之氣血流通不平衡，產生了左右溫差。

根據人體動則生熱的規律，確定體溫低的右邊，就是氣血不通的所在。所以我們就將ＸＨ治療儀的電波，主要輸入到發冷一側上下肢體的主要穴位和神經，僅經一次治療，就產生明顯的治療效果，經過３２天治療，症狀就全部消除，病人病痛已一年二個月了，至今身體仍然很健康。此病用西醫又從何入手醫治呢？

"坐起來就要倒下的人"之攻克

這個病例從中醫角度來看，主要是控制坐姿的神經和部位，發生病變，也就是氣血不通，祇要使這些部位的電阻，電容，電導值，恢復正常，就能消除症狀。

所以我們就把ＸＨ治療儀的電波，輸入到有關的神經與部位，僅治療一個小時病人就恢復健康，病人試著躺下，然後自己坐起來，連續三次，均很正常，這位病人，從治癒到現在，已經快滿十個多月了，現在身體仍然很健康。此病用西醫又從何入手醫治呢？

"右腳失去知覺的人"之攻克

這個病例從中醫角度來看，那裡有病痛，就是那裡發生了氣血不通，那麼對ＸＨ療法而言，制定治療方案就太簡單了。我們把ＸＨ治療儀的電波，通過大面積的網狀電極，施加於右腳的腿部和踝部，僅一次治療，病人就基本恢復知覺，經二次治療，右腳對痛覺的反應與正常的左腳就一樣了，症狀完全消除，恢復正常。病人病痛已六個多月了，至今右腳仍很正常。此病用西醫又從何入手醫治呢？

中醫的氣血論值得重視

根據上述病例分析，證明世界上有些病，用西醫是無法解釋，也是無法醫治的。用中醫的氣血論確可解釋，從氣血論入手，使用ＸＨ療法，有些病卻是很容易醫治，並能使病痛很快地減輕或消除。

頸椎的骨質增生物到那裡去了呢？

當然有些病例用氣血論可解釋，確無法用現代科學來說明其所以然。

四年多來，我們收治頸椎骨質增生的患者共有３１例，這種病人頭頸強直，頭部無法左右轉動，如欲觀看左右景物，人也必須全身隨著左右轉動。

根據氣血論，那裡病痛，那裡就是氣血不通，頸部強直，使頭部不能左右轉動，那麼必然是頸部發生氣血不通。根據ＸＨ療法的治療要點，理所當然的，應將電波輸入病變部位——頸部。結果奇蹟出現了，絕大部份患者，在１４天至３２天，消除症狀，去醫院復查，從頸椎的Ｘ光片中，再也看不到病變的情況了，那麼骨質增生物到那裡去了呢？

奇蹟每天在發生

這樣的奇蹟，每天都在曼谷第十二戒毒所門診部發生，四年多來慕名而來，要求用ＸＨ療法治病和戒毒者，共達六萬多人次以上，尤其是那些查無病因的怪病，及某些疑難雜症，用ＸＨ療法，療效達９５％以上，用於戒毒，療效更是高達９９％以上。

ＸＨ療法對下列廿種病，具有９５％以上的治療效果：

１．心臟病；２．高血壓；３．低血壓；４．頭痛；５．偏頭痛；６．頭暈；７．美尼爾氏症；８．青光眼；９．失眠；１０．頭頸痛；１１．落枕；１２．過敏性鼻炎；１３．扭挫傷；１４．腰背酸痛；１５．關節痛；１６．關節水腫；１７．胃病；１８．嘔吐；１９．月經痛；２０．查無病因的怪病；２１．走火入魔。

ＸＨ療法，對消除或減輕因海洛英等毒癮嚴重發作而引起的下列十七種病苦具有９９％以上的治療效果：

１．頭痛；２．頭暈；３．欲睡；４．打哈欠；５．打噴嚏；６．頭頸痛；７．背脊痛；８．腰痛；９．手腳肌肉痠痛；１０．肚痛；１１．內臟痙攣痛；１２．嘔吐；１３．胸悶；１４．胸痛；１５．心悸、心速；１６．手腳發冷、全身出冷汗；１７．無力。

非病情重者不收

由於本所ＸＨ治療機缺乏，現在每天最多祇能收治１２８人，目前主要收治戒毒者，因為毒品對社會的安全影響太大。

其他病患，政府規定，必須是各大醫院查無病因，病情很重，又無法醫治者，我醫務所才能根據病情，限額收治。目前政府正在設法解決問題，使ＸＨ療法擴展到更多的醫務所和醫院，到時泰國地區，一定能滿足更多的病患者之要求。

ＤＲ．ＹＡＮ ＬＡＩＹＩＮ晏萊蔭博士
泰國曼谷市衛生廳專家醫師
一九九一年十月一日寫於曼谷
TEL:(662)5851672, 5885068
FAX:(662)5885068

Clinical Experimental Report on Using XH-1 to Treat Drug Addiction on 100 Heroin Quitters by the 12th Narcotic Clinic (19th Medical Clinic), Bangkok Metropolitan Administration

Person in Charge of the Experiment

Dr. Kachit Choopanya   President of Department of Health, Bangkok Metropolitan Administration.

Principal Investigator

Dr. Laiyin Yan   Specialized physician for drug-addiction treatment of Department of Health, Bangkok Metropolitan Administration and the inventor of XH-1 illness and drug-addiction therapy.

Participants of the Experiment

Dr. Suphak Vanichseni   Vice-president of Department of Health, Bangkok Metropolitan Administration.

Dr. Suwanee Raktham   Person in charge of the Drug Prevention and Treatment Center, Bangkok Metropolitan Administration.

Ms. Suneeporn Anuttarakulvanich   Person in charge of the Anuttarakulvanich Twelfth Narcotic Clinic, Bangkok Metropolitan Administration.

Mrs. Monta Tansuhuch   Nurse in charge of the Twelfth Narcotic Clinic, Bangkok Metropolitan Administration.

Content of the Experiment

1) Route Used for the Drug-Addiction Treatment.
2) Purpose of the Experiment.
3) Technical Demand of the Experiment.
4) Illness and Drug-Addiction Therapy.
5) Demand and Analysis on Selecting Participating Drug Quitters.
6) Experimental Report on Drug-Addiction Treatment.
7) Experimental Report on Health-Recovery Treatment.
8) Summary.

Route Used for the Drug-Addiction Treatment.

Adopting Dr. Laiyin Yan's drug-addiction therapy. Using XH-1's small electrical current, invented by Dr. Laiyin Yan, to treat illnesses as the method to treat drug addiction.

Purpose of the Experiment.

Observing the effect of treating heroin addiction using XH-1.

I. Observing, when heroin quitters' withdrawal reacts, XH-1 illnesses and drug-addiction therapy's relieving conditions of the seventeen withdrawal symptoms produced.

II. Observing whether XH-1 illness and drug-addiction therapy can effectively suppress heroin quitters' usual climax of the severe withdrawal reaction of the third and fourth days.

III. Observing any presence of special phenomenon during the whole course of drug-addiction treatment.

IV. Observing, after the XH-1 health-recovery treatment, the rehabilitating conditions of heroin users' six worst items of health condition.

I. Observing, When Heroin Quitters' Withdrawal Reacts, XH-1 Illnesses and Drug-Addiction Therapy's Relieving Conditions of the Seventeen Withdrawal Symptoms Produced.

    A. Heroin quitters' seventeen withdrawal symptoms:1) headache, 2) dizziness, 3) drowsiness, 4) yawning, 5) sneezing, 6) neck pain, 7) back and spinal pain, 8) lumbar pain, 9) muscle cramp of limbs, 10) abdominal pain, 11) cramp of internal organs, 12) nausea, 13) tight chest, 14) chest pain, 15) palpitation, 16) cold sweat with cold hands and feet, and 17) weakness.

    B. Observing each subject's daily conditions of drug-addiction treatment. Everyday each heroin quitter who comes to receive XH-1 illness and drug-addiction therapy must fill out a "Statistical Chart of Each Subject's Daily Therapeutic Effect of Drug-Addiction Treatment" (Chart 1-A).

        1. Observing, before receiving the daily XH-1 drug-addiction treatment, what are the withdrawal symptoms heroin quitters' have. Represent each of the three degree types of withdrawal symptom by "heavy," "medium," and "light."

        2. Observing, after receiving the daily thirty minutes of XH-1 drug-addiction treatment, the therapeutic effect on heroin quitters' withdrawal symptoms. Represent the condition types by "conspicuously effective," "effective," and "not effective."

        3. Increase the frequency of the required urine test to observe and see if there are subjects going back to use the drug again, such as if urine test shows drug positive, and list them as drug re-users and as the failure part of drug-addiction treatment.

    C. Observing the daily total condition of drug-addiction treatment: According to data "Statistical Chart of Each Subject's Daily Therapeutic Effect of Drug-Addiction Treatment" (Chart 1-A), construct "Statistical Chart of the Daily Total Condition of Drug-Addiction Treatment" (Chart 2), (2-1) to (2-7).

        1. Observing, before receiving the daily XH-1 drug-addiction treatment, heroin quitters' total number of types of degree of severity of withdrawal symptoms and the group population change of each withdrawal symptom. Represent the three degrees of severity of the symptoms by "severe," "medium," and "light."

        2. Observing, after receiving the daily thirty minutes of XH-1 illness and drug-addiction treatment, the total therapeutic effect on heroin quitters' symptoms and the condition of the group population. Represent the therapeutic effect on the symptoms

by "conspicuously effective," "effective," and "not effective."
D. Observing, during the seven-day course of drug-addiction treatment, XH-1's therapeutic effect on each of the seventeen withdrawal symptoms.
1. According to data "group population of the daily degrees of severity of each withdrawal symptom" from data in "Statistical Chart of the Daily Total Condition of Drug-Addiction Treatment" (Chart 2), construct "Graph of the Therapeutic Effect on Withdrawal Symptoms" (Chart 3), (3-1) to (3-15).
2. Analyze the daily group population-change curve of the degrees of severity. Analyze, during the seven-day course of XH-1 drug-addiction treatment, the condition of daily increase, decrease, and elimination of the total group population of the degrees of severity of each withdrawal symptom to assure XH-1's therapeutic effect on each withdrawal symptom.

II. Observing Whether XH-1 Illness and Drug-Addiction Therapy Can Effectively Suppress Heroin Quitters' Usual Climax of the Severe Withdrawal Reaction of the Third and Fourth Days.
A. Observing, during the course of drug-addiction treatment, whether the number of types of each subject's daily average withdrawal symptoms has a tendency to increase or decrease, to assure if XH-1 can effectively suppress heroin quitters' usual climax of the severe withdrawal reaction of the third and fourth days.
1. According to data in the "Statistical Chart of the Daily Total Condition of Drug-Addiction Treatment" (Chart 2), statistically calculate: the daily total group population of heroin quitters' withdrawal symptoms.
2. Also calculate: the daily average number of types of withdrawal symptoms per person.
3. Construct: "Graph of Daily Average Number of Types of Withdrawal Symptoms Per Person" (Chart 4).
B. Observing, during the course of drug-addiction treatment, whether the total group population change of the three degrees of severity of heroin quitters' withdrawal symptoms has a tendency to increase or decrease in order to assure if XH-1 can effectively suppress heroin quitters' usual climax of the severe withdrawal reaction of the third and fourth days.
1. According to data in the "Statistical Chart of the Daily Total Condition of Drug-Addiction Treatment" (Chart 2), statistically calculate: the total subjects' (group population's) daily degrees of severity of symptoms.
2. Construct: "Graph of the Total Subjects' Daily Changes of the

Degrees of Severity of Symptoms" (Chart 5).

III. Observing Any Presence of Special Phenomenon during the Whole Course of Drug-Addiction Treatment.
    A. During the seven-day course of drug-addiction treatment, each heroin quitter's condition of drug-addiction treatment must be strictly supervised for any special phenomenon.
    B. Special phenomenon should include the following: 1) physiological, 2) psychological, 3) any adverse effect, 4) any medical incident, 5) any good condition, 6) any bad condition, and 7) any safety/security incident.
    C. If there is any presence of special phenomenon, whether it is large or small, it should be reported immediately to the person in charge of this project, have a consultation meeting to analyze the condition and decide any of the following:
        1. Adopt certain types of safety security action.
        2. How to improve the drug-addiction treating techniques.
        3. Whether the therapy should continue.
        4. Whether the therapy should temporarily cease.
    D. If there is any presence of special phenomenon, it should be recorded into the "Statistical Chart of the Daily Total Condition of Drug-Addiction Treatment" (Chart 2). If there is a high daily group population of special phenomenon, then it must be shown by constructing the "Graph of Special Phenomenon during the Course of Drug-Addiction Treatment" (Chart 10).

IV. Observing and Analyzing over the Seven-Day Course of Drug-Addiction Treatment Items of Analysis and Statistics of Analyzing the Total Group Population and Condition of the Relieving Effect of Withdrawal Symptoms Using XH-1 Illness and Drug-Addiction Therapy
    A. Group population of drug-addiction treatment participants.
    B. Group population of those with withdrawal symptoms successfully relieved.
    C. Group population of those who failed.
    D. Investigation and analysis of reasons for failing.

V. Observing, after the XH-1 Health-Recovery Treatment, the Rehabilitating Conditions of Heroin Users' Six Worst Items of Health Condition.
    A. Heroin users' six worst items of health condition: 1. food appetite, 2. sleep, 3. spirited feel after awakening, 4. physical strength, 5. degree of comfort symptom, and 6. sexual appetite.
    B. Observing the condition of each subject's daily health-recovery treatment:

1. When each health-recovery-treated person receives XH-1 treatment daily, he (or she) must fill out a "Statistical Chart of Each Subject's Daily Rehabilitating Degree" (Chart 1-B).
2. Observing the health condition of the six health items of subjects receiving the XH-1 health-recovery treatment daily. The health condition is represented by: "good," "fair," and "poor."
3. Increase the frequency of the required urine test to observe and see if there are subjects going back to use drugs again, such as if the urine test shows drug positive, and list them as drug re-users and as the failure part of drug-addiction treatment.

C. According to data "Statistical Chart of Each Subject's Daily Rehabilitating Degree" (Chart 1-B), analyze and statistically calculate the total group population's daily rehabilitating degree of the health items. Construct "The Daily Statistical Chart of the Total Group Population's Rehabilitating Degree of Health Items" (Chart 6), (6-1) to (6-7).

D. According to data in "The Daily Statistical Chart of the Total Group Population's Rehabilitating Degree of Health Items" (Chart 6), analyze and statistically calculate the group population's daily changing tendency of "good," "fair," and "poor" of each of the heroin quitters' health items during the seven-day course of health-recovery treatment using XH-1. Construct the "Graph of the Group Population's Daily Changing Tendency of Health Items in Terms of Good, Fair, and Poor" (Chart 7), (7-1) to (7-6).

E. According to data in "The Daily Statistical Chart of the Total Group Population's Rehabilitating Degree of Health Items" (Chart 6), analyze and statistically calculate the total group population's daily changing tendency of total health items in terms of "good," "fair," and "poor" during the seven-day course of health-recovery treatment using XH-1. Construct "Graph of Total Group Population's Daily Changing Tendency of the Total Health Items in Terms of Good, Fair, and Poor" (Chart 8).

F. According to data in "The Daily Statistical Chart of the Total Group Population's Rehabilitating Degree of Health Items" (Chart 6), analyze and statistically calculate, after the seven-day course of health-recovery treatment, XH-1's rehabilitating effect on each of heroin users' six worst items of health condition on the last day (seventh day) in terms of "good," "fair," and "poor."

G. According to data in "The Daily Statistical Chart of the Total Group Population's Rehabilitating Degree of Health Items" (Chart 6), analyze and statistically calculate, after the seven-day course of health-recovery treatment, XH-1's total rehabilitation effect on heroin users' six worst items of health condition in percentage form of those who really participated the health-recovery treatment.

H. Observing, during the seven-day course of health-recovery treatment, whether there is anyone with withdrawal reaction.

1. Represent by constructing the "Statistical Chart of the Group Population's Daily Number of Types of Daily Withdrawal Symptoms during the Course of Health-Recovery Treatment" (Chart 9).

2. If there are people with withdrawal symptom, calculate them as the failure part quitting drugs.

Illness and Drug-Addiction Therapy.

I. Therapeutic Locations to Place the XH-1 Electrodes for Drug-Addiction Treatment:

A. Location J pairs with Location N

B. Location Z pairs with Location N (or the skin surface of painful/discomfort points)

II. Therapeutic Locations to Place the XH-1 Electrodes for Health-Recovery Treatment:

A. Location J pairs with Location N

B. Location Z pairs with Location S

For photographic illustration of the therapeutic locations, see Page 136.

III. The Whole Course of Drug-Addiction Treatment: The whole course of drug-addiction treatment is divided into two courses of treatments: drug-addiction treatment and health-recovery treatment.

A. Course of drug-addiction treatment: once per day, thirty minutes each time, continue for seven days.

B. Course of health-recovery treatment: once per day, thirty minutes each time, continue for seven days.

IV. Rules for the Usage of XH-1 Rehabilitation Therapeutic Machine:

A. Place the XH-1 electrodes on the drug quitters' skin surface of the related and painful/discomfort locations.

B. Between the skin surface and the electrodes, fill in a 1.2 cm. area of tap-water moistened eight-layer paper towel for isolation. The purpose of isolation is to prevent skin contamination: Dispose the paper towel after use.

C.There is no positive or negative difference between the electrodes.

D.Use household tapes to hold the electrodes.

E.Control the output dial to the extent so that the drug quitter feels comfortable.

F. XH-1 sends out about one pulse per second. Each pulse lasts a few milliseconds long. If two AA batteries (DC 3 volt) are used as the power source, XH-1 can operate for one year and two months at the rate of two hours of usage per day. Therefore XH-1 is not just thrifty on electricity but also very safe. However using batteries to run XH-1 for an extended period of time can change the output wave shape and affect its therapeutic effect. Therefore it is recommended to use AC as the power source, because XH-1 can convert AC power into an extremely stable form of DC 3 volt, allows the output wave shape to not change, and allows the therapeutic effect to be raised.

Demand and Analysis on Selecting Participating Drug Quitters.

I.Demand on Selecting Participating Drug Quitters.

    A.Number of participants: 100

    B.Selecting drug-quitting subjects.

        1.Voluntary drug quitters.

        2.Participants must not have had other drug-addiction treatment for quitting drug this time.

        3.Drug-addiction treatment participants must not carry other diseases.

        4.Duration of heroin usage must be between one to two years.

        5.Age range: Seventeen to twenty-five years old.

II.Analysis on Participating Drug Quitters for This Time.

    A.Group population of participants-100 subjects. There were 92 males and 8 females sent by their parents to quit drugs.

    B.Age range: Seventeen to twenty-five years old.

    C.Duration of heroin usage ranges from no less than one-year to no more than three years.

    D.The health condition, except symptoms due to heroin usage, does not include other diseases.

    E.Drug quitters must not have had other drug-addiction treatment for quitting drug this time.

III.Analysis on the Reasons for the Drug-Quitting Participants' Failure of Quitting Drugs from the Past.

A. Out of the 100 drug quitters, 98 of them had tried other methods to quit drugs.

    1. Eleven of them used methadone.

    2. Eighty-seven of them used analgesics or hypnotics to substitute heroin.

B. For the eleven subjects who used Methadone drug-addiction therapy, investigate the reasons for failing.

    1. Four of them could not stand the withdrawal reactions on the third day of quitting the drug and reused the drug.

    2. Five of them, due to the addiction produced from Methadone, must come to narcotic clinic to drink Methadone daily, and commuting time of forty-five minutes to about an hour is too much of a hassle so they would rather go back to the drug.

    3. Two of the drug quitters were forced by the drug sellers to retake drug.

C. For the eighty-seven of the drug quitters who used analgesics or hypnotics to substitute heroin, investigate reasons for failing. Fourteen of the drug quitters retook the drug after not being able to stand the withdrawal reactions on the second-day morning after quitting drugs. Seventy-two of the drug quitters retook the drug after not being able to stand the withdrawal reactions on the third-day morning after quitting drugs. One of the drug quitters retook the drug after not being able to stand the withdrawal reactions on the third-day evening after quitting drugs.

D. Investigate reasons for failing by using Methadone drug-addiction therapy. Methadone is also a kind of drug, only the toxicity is not quite as severe, but it is also addictive and not easy to quit. The principle of using Methadone to treat drug addiction is simply using a less-toxic drug to substitute for the more toxic heroin. Therefore some drug quitters are not satisfied with Methadone drug-addiction therapy.

E. Analyze reasons for failing to quit drugs by using analgesics or hypnotics to substitute heroin. The main reason for failing is that drug quitters could not stand the usual climax of the severe withdrawal reaction of the third and fourth days; therefore, they failed to quit drugs.

F. Regardless of which method is used to treat heroin drug addiction, when heroin quitters' withdrawal reacts, whether the seventeen withdrawal symptoms produced can be relieved immediately and effectively suppress the usual climax of the severe withdrawal reaction of the third and fourth days is one of the most vital key problems of success and failing of treating heroin addiction. Of course there are also problems of psychotherapy, society, etc.

Experimental Report on Drug-Addiction Treatment.

I.Types and Characteristics of Heroin Quitters' Symptoms of Withdrawal Reaction during the Seven-Day Course of XH-1 Drug-Addiction Treatment. According to data in the "Statistical Chart of the Daily Total Condition of Drug-Addiction Treatment" (Chart 2):

A.Only fifteen symptoms of the withdrawal reaction appeared: 1) headache, 2) dizziness, 3) drowsiness, 4) yawning, 5) sneezing, 6) neck pain, 7) back and spinal pain, 8) lumbar pain, 9) muscle cramp of limbs, 10) abdominal pain, 11) nausea, 12) tight chest, 13) palpitation, 14) cold sweat with cold hands and feet, and 15) weakness.

B.Symptoms which did not appear are: 1) chest pain and 2) cramp of internal organs.

C.Characteristics of the withdrawal symptoms: According to the analysis and statistics of data in the "Graph of the Therapeutic Effect on Withdrawal Symptoms" (Chart 3), heroin quitters' characteristics of the withdrawal symptoms are:

1.First day, mainly drowsiness.

2.Second day, both drowsiness and pain.

3.Third and fourth days, mainly pain.

4.Fifth and sixth days, health condition recovers.

5.From first day to sixth day, neck pain, back/spinal pain, heart palpitation, and weakness all exist.

D.During the seven-day course of drug-addiction treatment, the degrees of severity of the above fifteen withdrawal symptoms all belong to medium and light levels; a heavy levels a of severity did not exist.

II.The Immediate Effect after Thirty Minutes of Treating Fifteen Types of Heroin Withdrawal Symptoms by Using XH-1 during the Seven-Day Course of Drug-Addiction Treatment. According to the analysis and statistics of data in the "Statistical Chart of the Daily Total Condition of Drug-Addiction Treatment" (Chart 2):

A.The total number of every subject's daily drug withdrawal symptom types is: Total = 267 + 224 + 214 + 151 + 45 + 16 + 3 = 920.

B.The total number of the group population's symptom types with conspicuous therapeutic effect is: Total = 201 + 202 + 208 + 143 + 42 + 14 + 1 = 811. 811/920 x 100 = 88.1% conspicuous therapeutic effect.

C.The total number of the group population's symptom types with therapeutic effect is: Total = 51 + 20 + 4 + 6 + 1 + 0 + 1 = 83. 83/920 x 100 = 9% therapeutic effect.

D.The total number of the group population's symptom types with no therapeutic effect is: Total = 15 + 2 + 2 + 2 + 2 + 2 + 1 = 26. 26/920 x 100 = 2.8% with no therapeutic effect.

E. XH-1's immediate therapeutic effect on fifteen heroin withdrawal symptoms after thirty minutes treatment is: 88.1% + 9% = 97.1%.

III. Therapeutic Effect after Treating Each of the Fifteen Types of Withdrawal Symptoms by Using XH-1 during the Seven-Day Course of Drug-Addiction Treatment. According to the analysis and statistics of data in the "Graph of the Therapeutic Effect on Withdrawal Symptoms" (Chart 3), XH-1 has conspicuous therapeutic effect on each of the fifteen withdrawal symptoms.

IV. Whether XH-1 Illness and Drug-Addiction Therapy Can Effectively Suppress Heroin Quitters' Usual Climax of the Severe Withdrawal Reaction of the Third and Fourth Days.

A. According to the analysis and statistics of data in the "Graph of Daily Average Number of Types of Withdrawal Symptoms Per Person" (Chart 4):

1. XH-1 drug-addiction therapy has a conspicuous therapeutic effect on reducing the number of types of withdrawal symptoms.

2. XH-1 drug-addiction therapy has a conspicuous suppressing effect on heroin quitters' usual climax of the severe withdrawal reaction of the third and fourth days.

B. According to the analysis and statistics of data in the "Graph of the Total Subjects' Daily Changes of the Degrees of Severity of Symptoms" (Chart 5), XH-1 drug-addiction treatment has a conspicuous suppressing effect on heroin quitters' usual climax of the severe withdrawal reaction of the third and fourth days.

V. Whether There Is Presence of Special Phenomenon During the Seven-Day Course of Drug-Addiction Treatment Using XH-1. According to the analysis and statistics of data in the "Graph of the Daily Group Population of Subjects who Crave for High Volume of Food" of "The Special Phenomenon during the Course of Drug-Addiction Treatment" (Chart 10), constructed according to the analysis and statistics of data in the "Statistical Chart of the Daily Total Condition of Drug-Addiction Treatment" (Chart 2), the numbers of subjects who crave for high volumes of food are: Fifth day: 11, Sixth day: 34, Seventh day: 54.

VI. The Total Group Population, Condition, and Effect of the Relief of Withdrawal Symptoms Using XH-1 Illness and Drug-Addiction Therapy during the Seven-Day Course of Drug-Addiction Treatment. According to the analysis and statistics of data in the "Statistical Chart of the Daily

Total Condition of Drug-Addiction Treatment" (Chart 2):

    A. Number of voluntary heroin-addiction treatment participants: 92 males, 8 females, total of 100 subjects.

    B. Number of subjects with the withdrawal successfully relieved is: 89 males, 5 females, total of 94 subjects. Success rate is 94 percent as the urine tests after the eighth day showed drug negative.

    C. Number of subjects failed to quit drug: 3 males, 3 females, total of 6 subjects. Failing rate is 6 percent.

    D. Investigate reasons for failing to quit drug:

        1. Subject 1: Name XXXX, male, age twenty-four. Number of drug-addiction treatments received: once, thirty minutes each time. Because he could not get a day off from work, he was not able to continue the drug-addiction treatment.

        2. Subject 2: Name XXXX, female, age eighteen. Number of drug-addiction treatments received: once, thirty minutes each time. Because she had to work and could not accept thirty minutes of drug-addiction treatment everyday, she switched to Methadone drug-addiction therapy.

        3. Subject 3: Name XXXX, male, age twenty-one. Number of drug-addiction treatments received: twice, thirty minutes each time. He could not stand the withdrawal reaction on the third-day morning, so he continued to take drugs.

        4. Subject 4: Name XXXX, female, age nineteen. Number of drug-addiction treatments received: three times, thirty minutes each time. Withdrawal reacted on the fourth-day morning, and she was not able to get off the bed, so she could not stand it and had to continue to take drugs.

        5. Subject 5: Name XXXX, male, age twenty-three. Number of drug-addiction treatments received: three times, thirty minutes each time. Withdrawal reacted on the fourth-day morning, and no one could take him to the narcotic clinic for drug-addiction treatment, so he could not stand it and had to continue to take drugs.

        6. Subject 6: Name XXXX, female, age nineteen. Number of drug-addiction treatments received: twice, thirty minutes each time. She received the drug-addiction treatment on the first day but not on the second day. Withdrawal reacted severely on the third-day morning, so she could not stand it and then came in for the second drug-addiction treatment. On the fourth-day morning, withdrawal reacted severely again, so she lost confidence and took drugs again.

Summary for the Above Reasons for Failing to Quit Drugs Includes the Following Three Points:

A.Subjects were not being able to stand heroin quitters' usual climax of the severe withdrawal reaction of the third and fourth days.

B.Due to having to work, subjects were not being able to receive the one-half hour drug-addiction treatment everyday.

C.Subjects do not have enough confidence to quit the drug.

Experimental Report on Health-Recovery Treatment.

I.Number of Health-Recovery Treatment Participants: 94

II.According to the Analysis of Data "Graph of the Group Population's Daily Changing Tendency of Health Items in Terms of Good, Fair, and Poor" (Chart 7), (7-1) to (7-6): During the seven-day course of health-recovery treatment using XH-1, heroin users' six worst items of health condition are: 1. food appetite, 2. sleep, 3. spirited feel after awakening, 4. physical strength, 5. degree of comfort symptom, and 6. sexual appetite.

III.According to the Analysis of Data "Graph of Total Group Population's Daily Changing Tendency of the Total Healthy Items in Terms of Good, Fair, and Poor" (Chart 8): During the seven-day health-recovery treatment using XH-1, the total "good" health items kept increasing daily. This is showing that XH-1 has a conspicuous rehabilitating effect on subjects who received health-recovery treatment.

IV. Health Conditions of the Ninety-four Patients Who Received Health-Recovery Treatment after Seven Days of XH-1 Health-Recovery Treatment. All subjects can eat well, sleep well, feel spirited after awakening and no longer have to stay in bed afterwards, have improved physical strength, and feel comfortable. Except two of the subjects, the rest of them also have improved sexual appetite.

V.Analyze and Statistically Calculate: The Rehabilitation and Therapeutic Effect of Each Health Item in Percentage Form Calculated by the Total Group Population Number of the Ninety-four Health-Recovery Treatment Participants, According to the Last Day's Data of "The Daily Statistical Chart of the Total Group Population's Rehabilitating Degree of Health Items" (Chart 6).

A.Food appetite (eating well): 94 with good degree of rehabilitation, efficacy rate 100%.

B.Sleep: 92 with good degree of rehabilitation, 2 with fair degree of

rehabilitation, efficacy rate 100%.
- C. Spirited feel after awakening: 92 with good degree of rehabilitation, 2 with fair degree of rehabilitation, efficacy rate 100%.
- D. Physical strength: 90 with good degree of rehabilitation, 4 with fair degree of rehabilitation, efficacy rate 100%.
- E. Degree of comfort symptom: 90 with good degree of rehabilitation, 4 with fair degree of rehabilitation, efficacy rate 100%.
- F. Sexual appetite: 83 with good degree of rehabilitation, 9 with fair degree of rehabilitation, 2 with poor degree of rehabilitation, efficacy rate 97.8%. Reason for having poor degree of rehabilitation on the 2 subjects is unknown.

VI. According to the Last Day's Data of "The Daily Statistical Chart of the Total Group Population's Rehabilitating Degree of Health Items" (Chart 6), Statistically Calculate XH-1'S Total Rehabilitation and Therapeutic Effect on the Six Worst Items of Health Condition in Percentage Form Calculated by the Total Group Population Number of the Ninety-four Health-Recovery Treatment Participants.
- A. Each item's group population is 94.
- B. Six items' group population = 94 x 6 = 564.
- C. Total group population of those with good degree of rehabilitation = 94 + 92 + 92 + 90 + 90 + 83 = 541. 541/564 x 100 = 95.9%.
- D. Total group population of those with fair degree of rehabilitation = 0 + 2 + 2 + 4 + 4 + 9 = 21. 21/564 x 100 = 3.7%.
- E. Total group population of those with poor degree of rehabilitation = 0 + 0 + 0 + 0 + 0 + 2 = 2. 2/564 x 100 = 0.4%.
- F. Total rehabilitating effect = 95.9% + 3.7% = 99.6%.

Summary

I. By using XH-1 to treat heroin drug addiction, heroin quitters' fifteen withdrawal symptoms can be relieved immediately after the thirty-minute drug-addiction treatment with an efficacy rate of 97.1%.

II. By using XH-1 to treat drug addiction, it can effectively suppress heroin quitters' usual climax of the severe withdrawal reaction of the third and fourth days.

III. By using XH-1 during the seven-day course of health-recovery treatment, some drug quitters appeared to have special phenomenon of cravings for food on the fifth to seventh days.

IV. The condition of using the XH-1 seven-day health-recovery treatment:
The rehabilitation efficacy rate of heroin quitters' six worst health items,
calculated by the total group population of ninety-four health-recovery
treatment participants, is 99.6%. The ninety-four health-recovery treatment participants, besides never having anymore withdrawal symptoms,
are able to eat well, sleep well, feel spirited after awakening and no longer
have to stay in bed afterwards, have improved physical strength, and
feel comfortable. Ninety-two of the subjects also have improved sexual
appetite.

V. The successful rate, in percentage form, of using XH-1 to treat heroin
addiction: Of the 100 heroin-addiction treatment participants, ninety-
four of them had their withdrawal symptoms relieved and had been rehabilitated successfully. According the urine test, it is proved that, during the "whole course" of fourteen days of drug-addiction treatment, all
94 drug quitters no longer took any more heroin. The successful rate of
drug-addiction treatment is 94 percent.

Dr. KACHIT CHOOPANYA
M.D., M.P.H., M.P.H. & T.M. (Tulane) U.S.A.
DEPUTY PERMANENT SECRETARY ON PUBLIC HEALTH
BANGKOK METROPOLITAN ADMINISTRATION

Date: Month: Year:

Name			Sex		Age		I.D. #	

Today's degree of severity of the withdrawal symptoms before the drug addiction treatment			Today's degree of severity of the withdrawal symptoms after the 30 minutes of drug addiction treatment			Today's degree of severity of the withdrawal symptoms before the drug addiction treatment			Today's degree of severity of the withdrawal symptoms after the 30 minutes of drug addiction treatment		
Withdrawal symptom	Degree of severity	Conspicuously effective	Effective	Not effective	Withdrawal symptom	Degree of severity	Conspicuously effective	Effective	Not effective		
dizziness	heavy				abdominal pain	heavy					
	medium					medium					
	light					light					
drowsiness	heavy				nausea	heavy					
	medium					medium					
	light					light					
yawning	heavy				palpitation	heavy					
	medium					medium					
	light					light					
sneezing	heavy				tight chest	heavy					
	medium					medium					
	light					light					
headache	heavy				neck pain	heavy					
	medium					medium					
	light					light					
back and spinal pain	heavy				weakness	heavy					
	medium					medium					
	light					light					
lumbar pain	heavy				cold sweat with cold hands and feet	heavy					
	medium					medium					
	light					light					
muscle cramp of limbs	heavy				chest pain	heavy					
	medium					medium					
	light					light					
cramp of internal organs	heavy				other						
	medium										
	light										

Date: Month: Year:

Name		Sex		Age		I.D. #	

Health Items	Health Condition		
	good	fair	poor
food appetite			
sleep			
spirited feel after awakening			
physical strength			
degree of comfort symptom			
sexual appetite			

(2-1)

STATISTICAL CHART OF THE DAILY TOTAL
CONDITION OF DRUG ADDICTION TREATMENT   No. of participants: 100

Group population of today's degree of severity of the withdrawal symptoms before the drug addiction treatment			Today's therapeutic effect after 30 minutes of treatment		
Symptom	Degree	Group population	# of subjects w/ conspicuous therapeutic effect	# of subjects with therapeutic effect	# of subjects with no therapeutic effect
dizziness	medium	57	50	7	0
	light	4	3	1	0
drowsiness	medium	42	8	25	9
	light	26	17	6	3
yawning	medium	28	20	7	1
sneezing	light	2	2	0	0
neck pain	medium	26	26	0	0
back and spinal pain	medium	17	17	0	0
	light	2	1	1	0
palpitation	medium	12	12	0	0
	light	3	3	0	0
weakness	medium	40	38	2	0
	light	8	4	2	2
Statistics	total	267	201	51	15
	medium, total	222	rate 75.3 %	rate 19.1 %	rate 5.6 %
	light, total	45			

267 / 100 = 2.67

Average # of symptoms per person is 2.67

〈2-2〉 part 1

STATISTICAL CHART OF THE DAILY TOTAL
CONDITION OF DRUG ADDICTION TREATMENT

No. of participants: 97

Group population of today's degree of severity of the withdrawal symptoms before the drug addiction treatment			Today's therapeutic effect after 30 minutes of treatment		
Symptom	Degree	Group population	# of subjects w/ conspicuous therapeutic effect	# of subjects with therapeutic effect	# of subjects with no therapeutic effect
dizzness	medium	17	16	1	0
	light	2	1	1	0
drowsiness	medium	15	11	4	0
	light	5	2	3	0
yawning	medium	3	2	1	0
headache	medium	8	8	0	0
	light	2	1	1	0
neck pain	medium	24	24	0	0
	light	4	4	0	0
back & spinal pain	medium	18	18	0	0
	light	6	4	2	0
lumbar pain	medium	8	7	1	0
	light	3	3	0	0

Statistical Chart of Each Subject's Daily Therapeutic Effect of Drug-Addiction Treatment (Chart 1-A)

Day 2

Chart 2

(2-2) part 2

STATISTICAL CHART OF THE DAILY TOTAL
CONDITION OF DRUG ADDICTION TREATMENT   No. of participants: **97**

Group population of today's degree of severity of the withdrawal symptoms before the drug addiction treatment			Today's therapeutic effect after 30 minutes of treatment		
Symptom	Degree	Group popu-lation	# of subjects w/ conspicuous therapeutic effect	# of subjects with therapeutic effect	# of subjects with no therapeutic effect
muscle cramp of limbs	medium	10	10	0	0
	light	8	7	1	0
abdominal pain	medium	3	3	0	0
nausea	medium	2	2	0	0
	light	1	1	0	0
palpitation	medium	21	21	0	0
	light	3	3	0	0
tight chest	medium	4	4	0	0
	light	1	1	0	0
weakness	medium	41	39	2	0
	light	15	10	3	2
Statistics	total	224	202	20	2
	medium, total	174	rate 90.2 %	rate 8.9 %	rate 0.9 %
	light, total	50			

224 / 97 = 2.3

Average # of symptoms per person is 2.3

79

STATISTICAL CHART OF THE DAILY TOTAL
CONDITION OF DRUG ADDICTION TREATMENT

No. of participants: 97

Group population of today's degree of severity of the withdrawal symptoms before the drug addiction treatment			Today's therapeutic effect after 30 minutes of treatment		
Symptom	Degree	Group popu-lation	# of subjects w/ conspicuous therapeutic effect	# of subjects with therapeutic effect	# of subjects with no therapeutic effect
headache	medium	11	11	0	0
	light	6	4	2	0
neck pain	medium	21	21	0	0
	light	18	18	0	0
back & spinal pain	medium	16	16	0	0
	light	9	8	1	0
lumbar pain	medium	8	8	0	0
	light	7	6	1	0
muscle cramp of limbs	medium	9	9	0	0
	light	9	9	0	0
abdominal pain	medium	2	2	0	0
	light	2	2	0	0
nausea	medium	2	2	0	0
	light	1	1	0	0

STATISTICAL CHART OF THE DAILY TOTAL
CONDITION OF DRUG ADDICTION TREATMENT

Chart 2

(2-3) part 2

No. of participants: 97

Group population of today's degree of severity of the withdrawal symptoms before the drug addiction treatment			Today's therapeutic effect after 30 minutes of treatment		
Symptom	Degree	Group population	# of subjects w/ conspicuous therapeutic effect	# of subjects with therapeutic effect	# of subjects with no therapeutic effect
palpitation	medium	23	23	0	0
	light	5	5	0	0
tight chest	medium	4	4	0	0
	light	3	3	0	0
cold sweat with cold hands & feet	medium	2	2	0	0
weakness	medium	41	41	0	0
	light	15	13	0	2
Statistics	total	214	208	4	2
	medium, total	139			
	light, total	75	rate 97.2 %	rate 1.9 %	rate 0.9 %

214 / 97 = 2.2

Average # of symptoms per person is   2.2

(**2-4**) part 1

STATISTICAL CHART OF THE DAILY TOTAL
CONDITION OF DRUG ADDICTION TREATMENT   No. of participants: **94**

Group population of today's degree of severity of the withdrawal symptoms before the drug addiction treatment			Today's therapeutic effect after 30 minutes of treatment		
Symptom	Degree	Group popu- lation	# of subjects w/ conspicuous therapeutic effect	# of subjects with therapeutic effect	# of subjects with no therapeutic effect
headache	medium	5	5	0	0
	light	8	6	2	0
neck pain	medium	11	11	0	0
	light	15	15	0	0
back and spinal pain	medium	9	9	0	0
	light	11	10	1	0
lumbar pain	medium	3	3	0	0
	light	6	5	1	0
muscle cramp of limbs	medium	2	2	0	0
	light	7	6	1	0
abdominal pain	light	2	1	1	0
nausea	light	1	1	0	0

STATISTICAL CHART OF THE DAILY TOTAL
CONDITION OF DRUG ADDICTION TREATMENT

No. of participants: 94

Group population of today's degree of severity of the withdrawal symptoms before the drug addiction treatment			Today's therapeutic effect after 30 minutes of treatment		
Symptom	Degree	Group popu-lation	# of subjects w/ conspicuous therapeutic effect	# of subjects with therapeutic effect	# of subjects with no therapeutic effect
palpitation	medium	16	16	0	0
	light	7	7	0	0
tight chest	light	2	2	0	0
weakness	medium	28	28	0	0
	light	18	16	0	2
Statistics	total	151	143	6	2
	medium, total	74			
	light, total	77	rate 94.7 %	rate 4.0 %	rate 1.3 %

151 / 94 = 1.6

Average # of symptoms per person is 1.6

STATISTICAL CHART OF THE DAILY TOTAL   (2-5)
CONDITION OF DRUG ADDICTION TREATMENT

No. of participants: 94

Group population of today's degree of severity of the withdrawal symptoms before the drug addiction treatment			Today's therapeutic effect after 30 minutes of treatment		
Symptom	Degree	Group popu-lation	# of subjects w/ conspicuous therapeutic effect	# of subjects with therapeutic effect	# of subjects with no therapeutic effect
headache	light	3	3	0	0
neck pain	light	6	6	0	0
back & spinal pain	light	5	5	0	0
lumbar pain	light	3	2	1	0
muscle cramp of limbs	light	3	3	0	0
palpitation	light	5	5	0	0
weakness	light	20	18	0	2
Statistics	total	45	42	1	2
	light, total	45	rate 93.3 %	rate 2.2 %	rate 4.4 %

45 / 94 = 0.48

Average # of symptoms per person is **0.48**
Special phenomenon: 11 subjects had craving for high volume of food.

Chart **2**

(2-6)

STATISTICAL CHART OF THE DAILY TOTAL
CONDITION OF DRUG ADDICTION TREATMENT

No. of participants: **94**

Group population of today's degree of severity of the withdrawal symptoms before the drug addiction treatment			Today's therapeutic effect after 30 minutes of treatment		
Symptom	Degree	Group popu-lation	# of subjects w/ conspicuous therapeutic effect	# of subjects with therapeutic effect	# of subjects with no therapeutic effect
neck pain	light	4	4	0	0
back & spinal pain	light	2	2	0	0
palpitation	light	3	3	0	0
weakness	light	7	5	0	2
Statistics	total	16	14	0	2
	light, total	16	rate 87.5 %	rate 0.0 %	rate 12.5 %

16 / 94 = 0.17

Average # of symptoms per person is 0.17

Special phenomenon: 34 subjects had craving for high volume of food.

(2-7)

STATISTICAL CHART OF THE DAILY TOTAL
CONDITION OF DRUG ADDICTION TREATMENT   No. of participants: **94**

Group population of today's degree of severity of the withdrawal symptoms before the drug addiction treatment			Today's therapeutic effect after 30 minutes of treatment		
Symptom	Degree	Group population	# of subjects w/ conspicuous therapeutic effect	# of subjects with therapeutic effect	# of subjects with no therapeutic effect
weakness	light	3	1	1	1
Statistics	total	3	1	1	1
	light, total	3	rate 33.3 %	rate 33.3 %	rate 33.3%

3 / 94 = 0.03

Average # of symptoms per person is 0.03

Special phenomenon: **54** subjects had craving for high volume of food.

86

GRAPH OF THE THERAPEUTIC EFFECT ON WITHDRAWAL SYMPTOMS

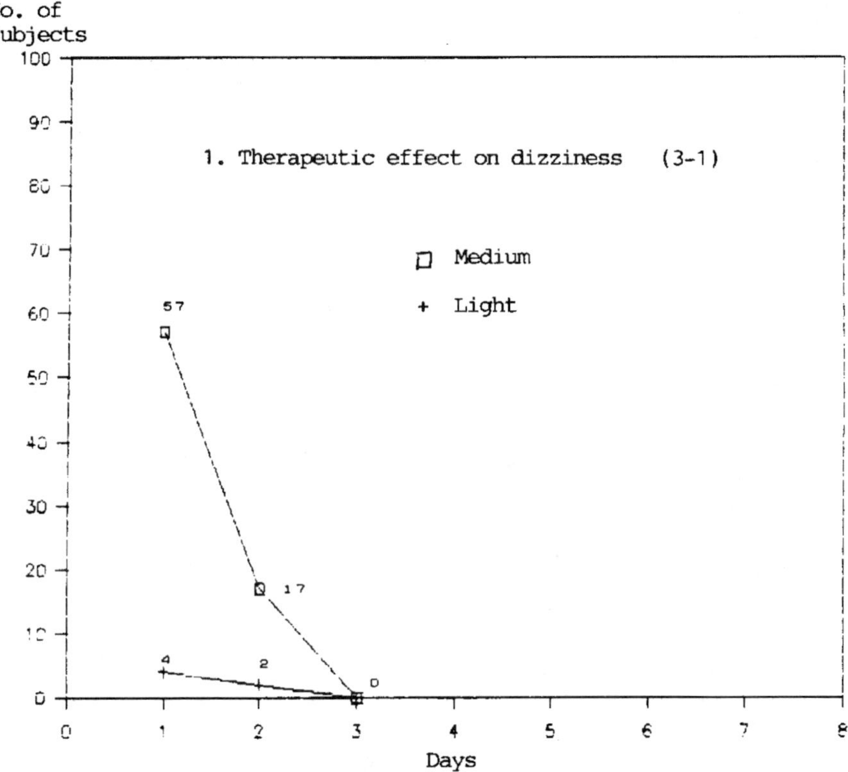

GRAPH OF THE THERAPEUTIC EFFECT ON WITHDRAWAL SYMPTOMS

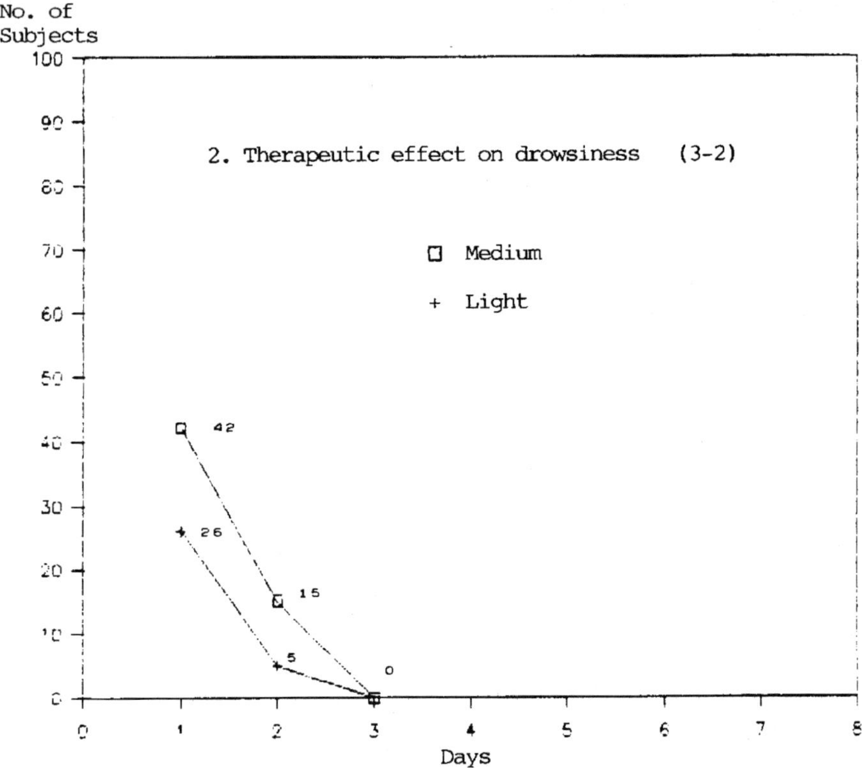

GRAPH OF THE THERAPEUTIC EFFECT ON WITHDRAWAL SYMPTOMS

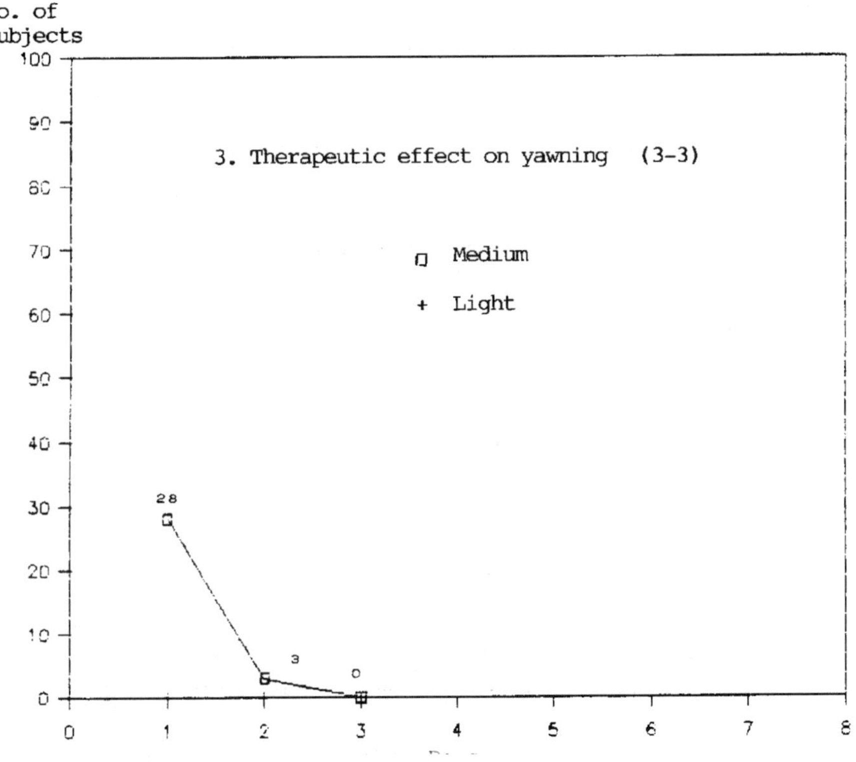

GRAPH OF THE THERAPEUTIC EFFECT ON WITHDRAWAL SYMPTOMS

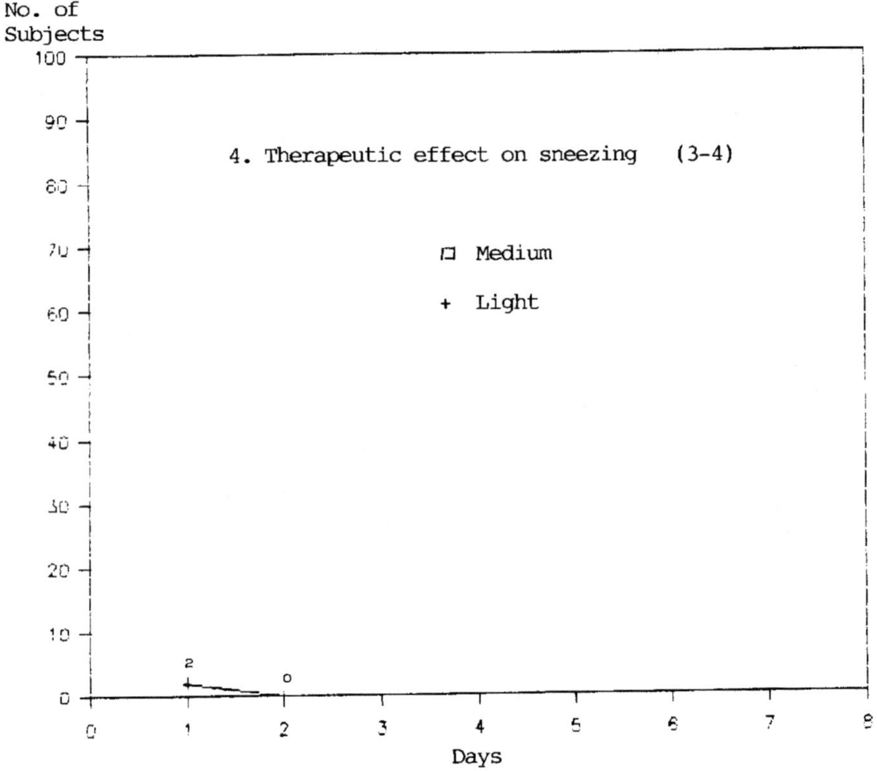

GRAPH OF THE THERAPEUTIC EFFECT ON WITHDRAWAL SYMPTOMS

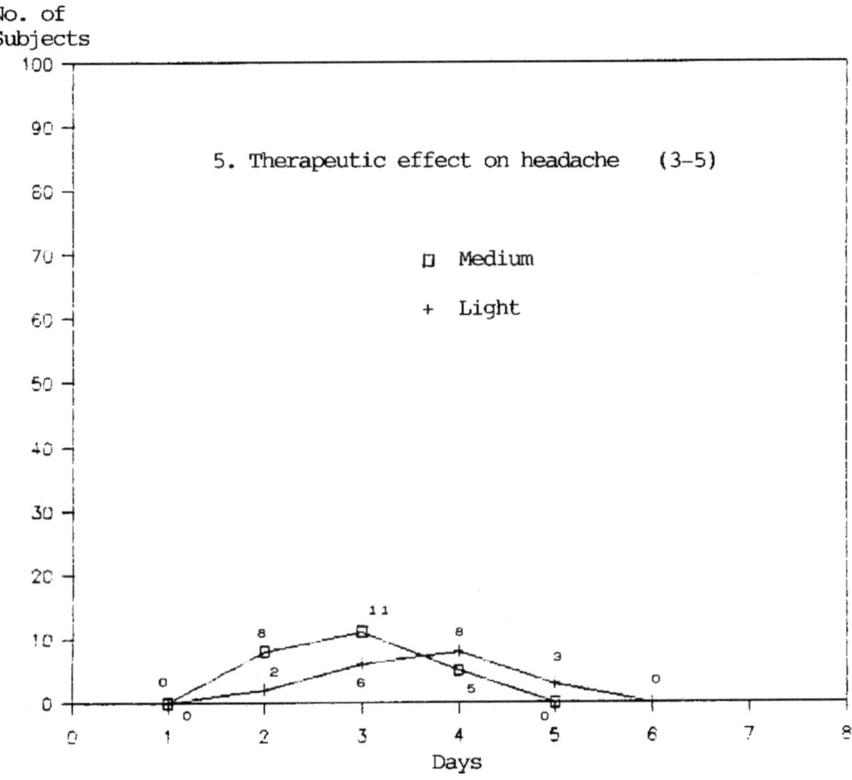

GRAPH OF THE THERAPEUTIC EFFECT ON WITHDRAWAL SYMPTOMS

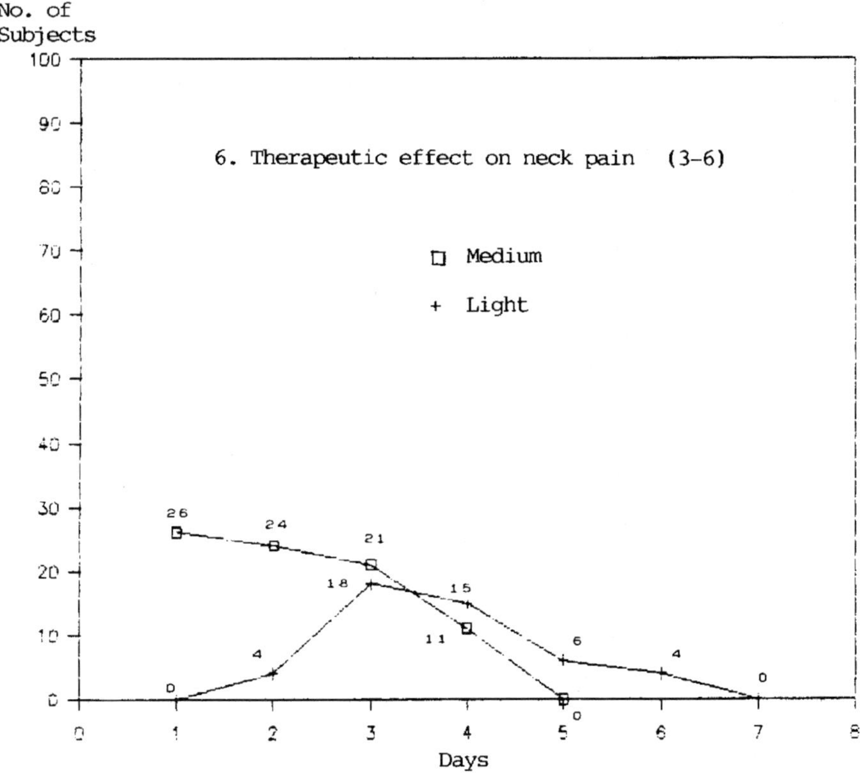

GRAPH OF THE THERAPEUTIC EFFECT ON WITHDRAWAL SYMPTOMS

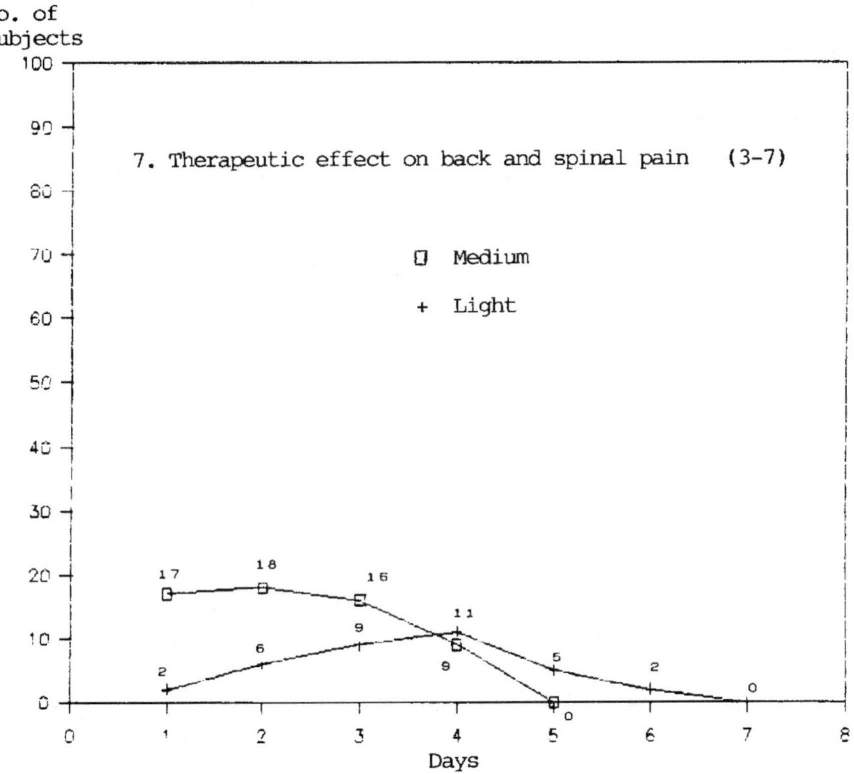

GRAPH OF THE THERAPEUTIC EFFECT ON WITHDRAWAL SYMPTOMS

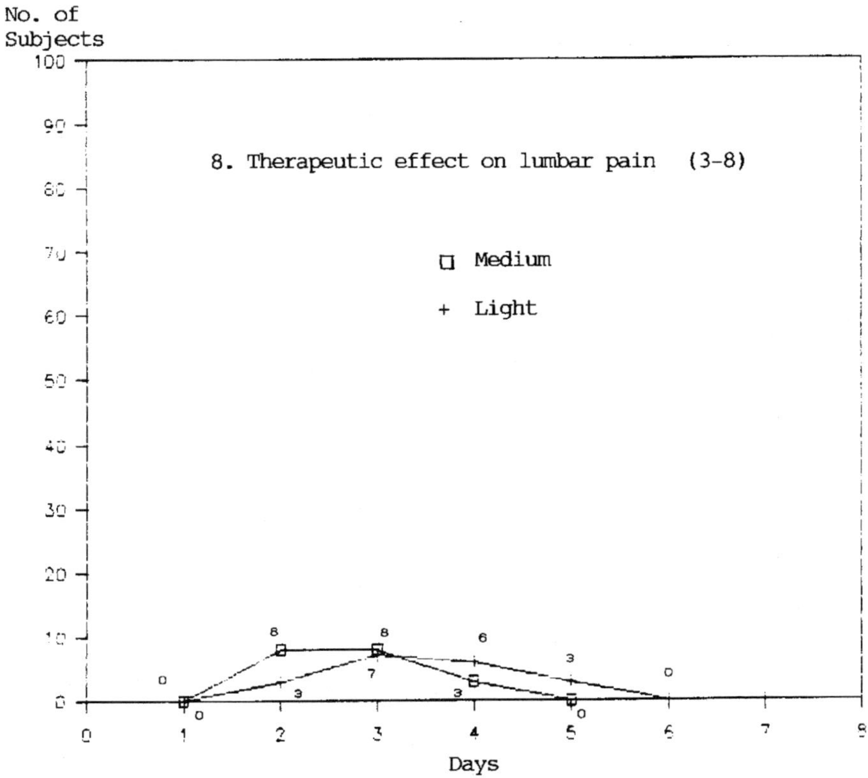

GRAPH OF THE THERAPEUTIC EFFECT ON WITHDRAWAL SYMPTOMS

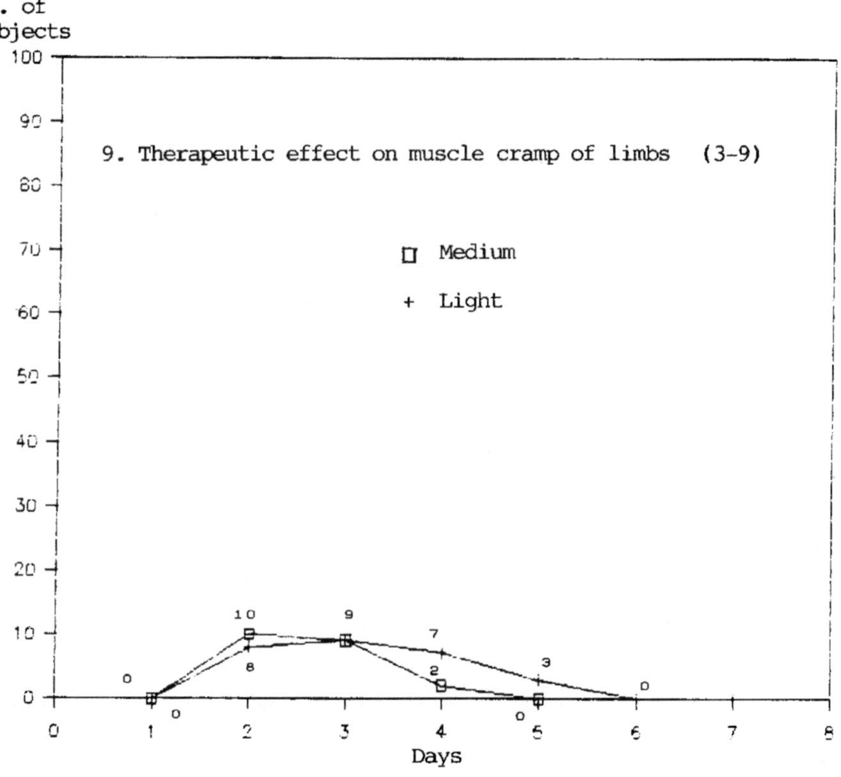

GRAPH OF THE THERAPEUTIC EFFECT ON WITHDRAWAL SYMPTOMS

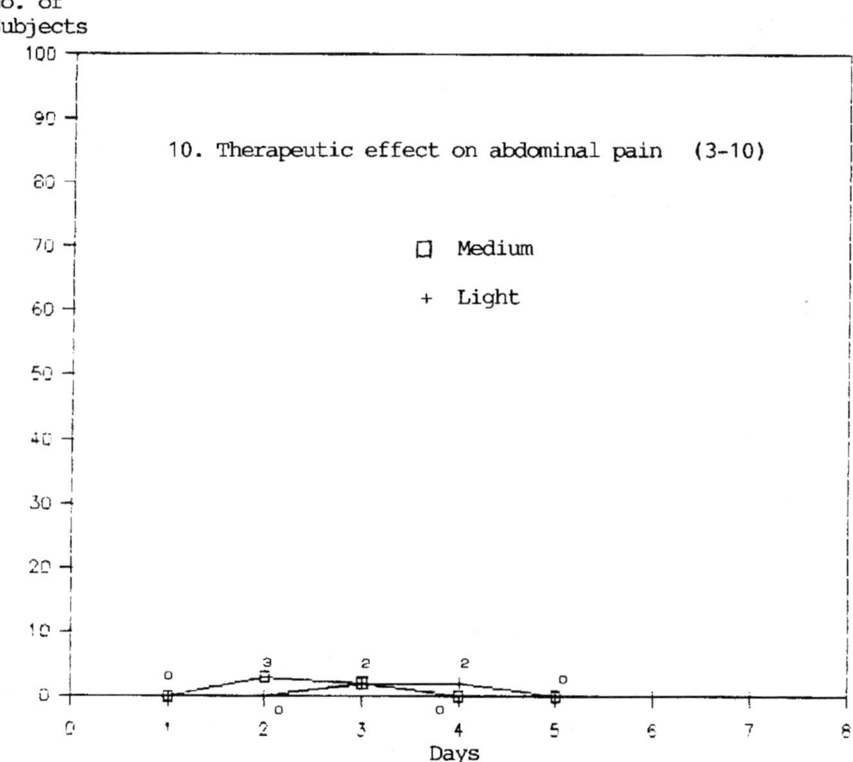

GRAPH OF THE THERAPEUTIC EFFECT ON WITHDRAWAL SYMPTOMS

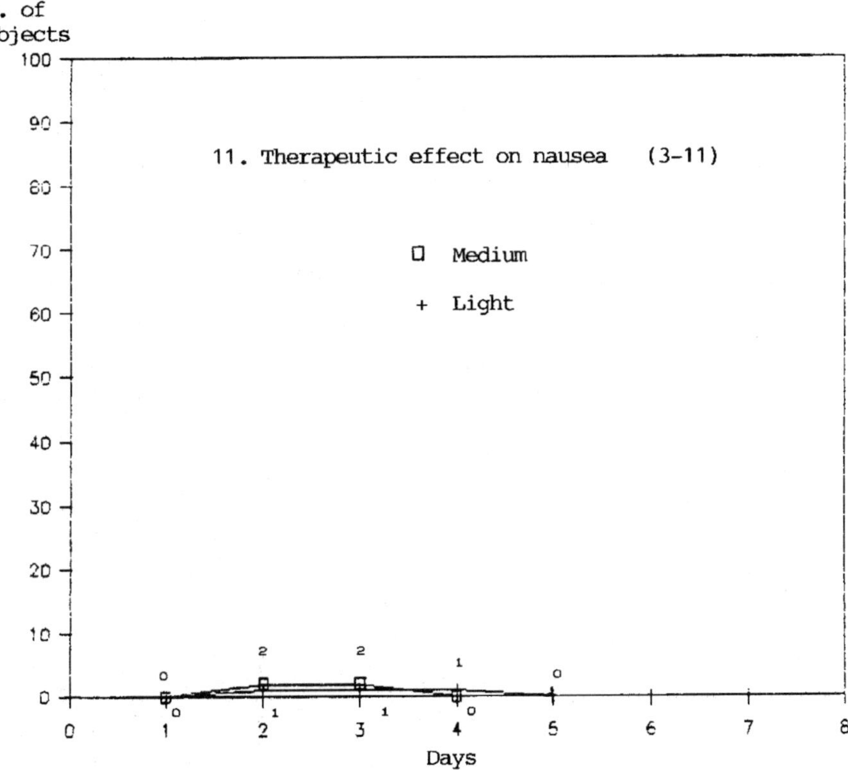

GRAPH OF THE THERAPEUTIC EFFECT ON WITHDRAWAL SYMPTOMS

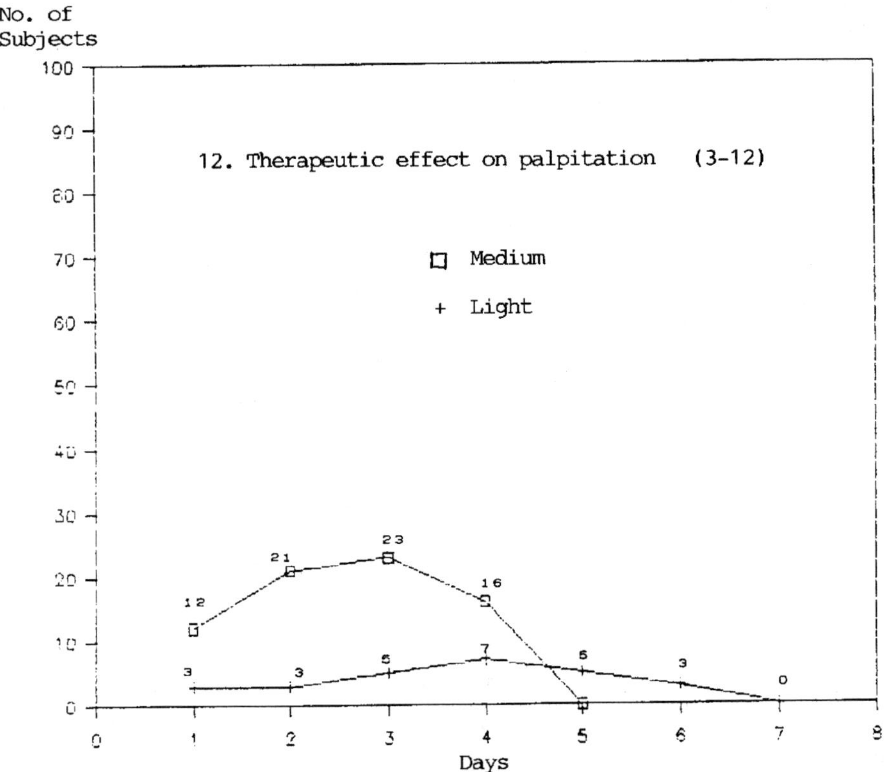

GRAPH OF THE THERAPEUTIC EFFECT ON WITHDRAWAL SYMPTOMS

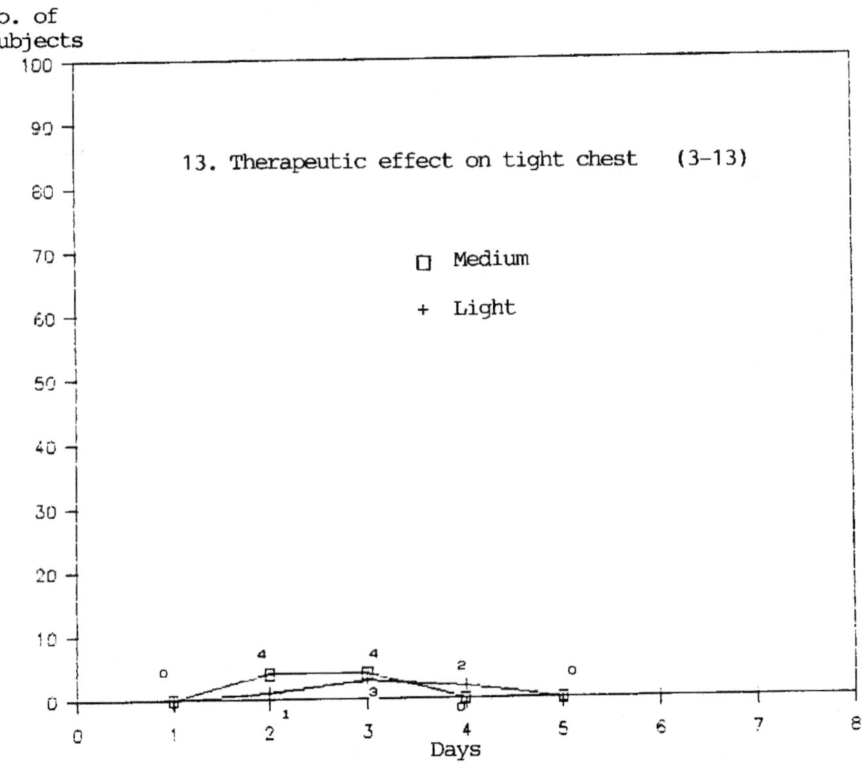

GRAPH OF THE THERAPEUTIC EFFECT ON WITHDRAWAL SYMPTOMS

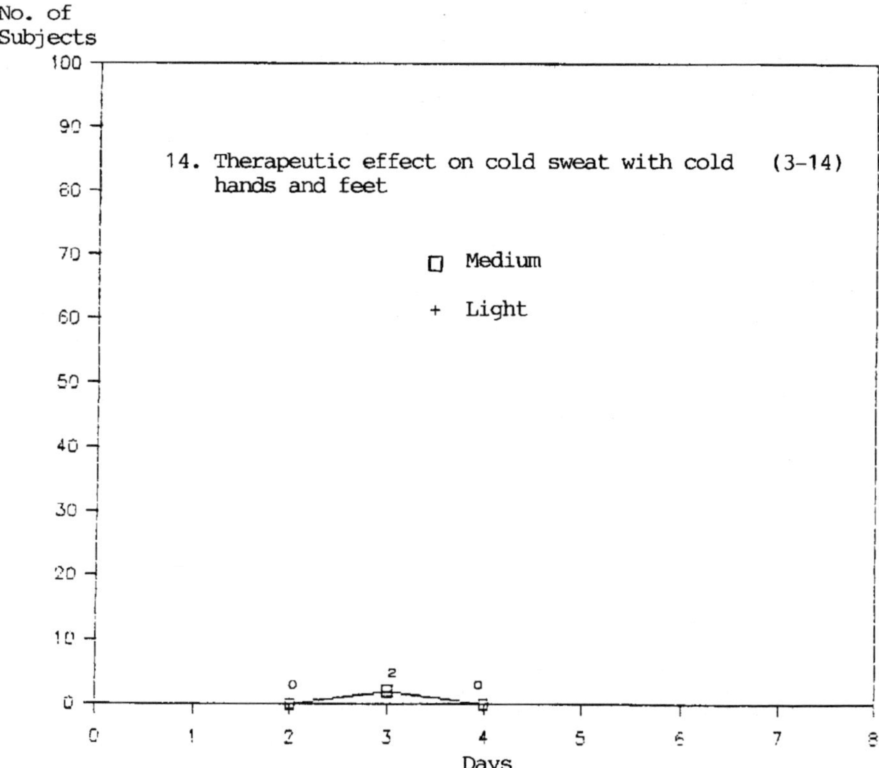

GRAPH OF THE THERAPEUTIC EFFECT ON WITHDRAWAL SYMPTOMS

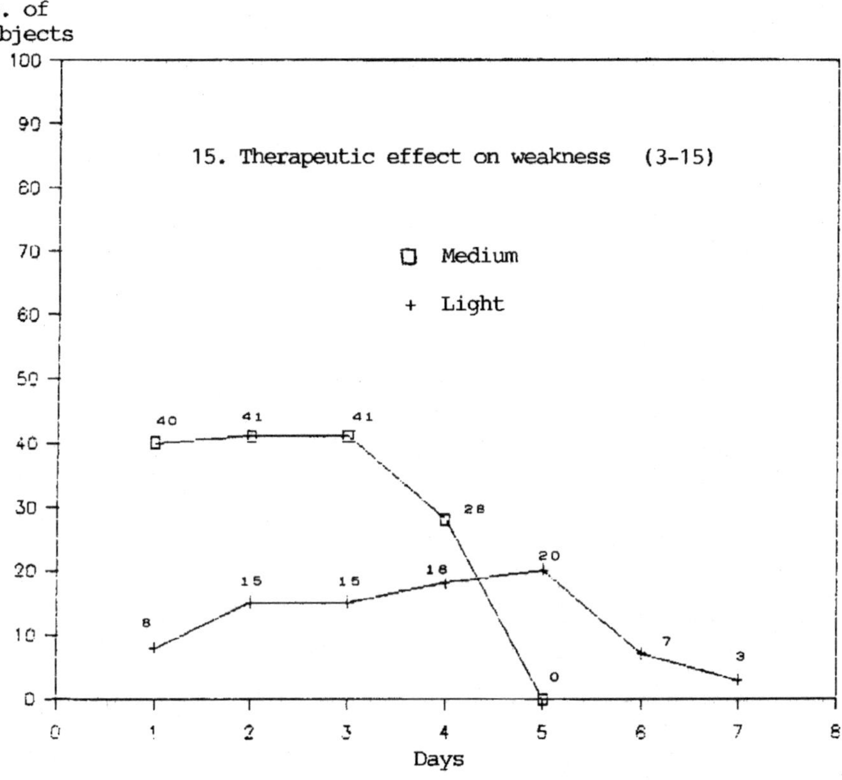

GRAPH OF THE DAILY AVERAGE NUMBER OF TYPES
OF WITHDRAWAL SYMPTOMS PER PERSON

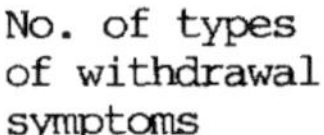

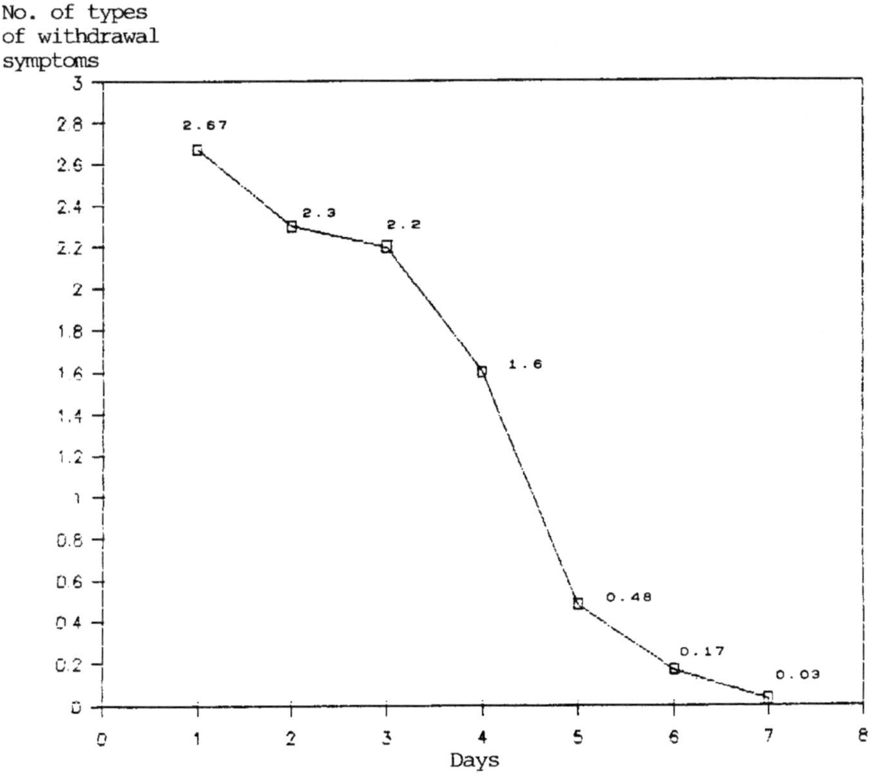

According to the analysis from the "graph of the daily average
number of types of withdrawal symptoms per person" constructed from
statistical data:

1. XH-1 drug addiction therapy has conspicuous therapeutic effect
on reducing the number of types of withdrawal symptoms.

2. XH-1 drug addiction therapy has conspicuous suppressing effect
on heroin quitters' severe withdrawal reaction of the 3rd and 4th day.

GRAPH OF THE TOTAL SUBJECTS' DAILY CHANGES
OF THE DEGREES OF SEVERITY OF SYMPTOMS

No. of all
subjects' total
symptoms

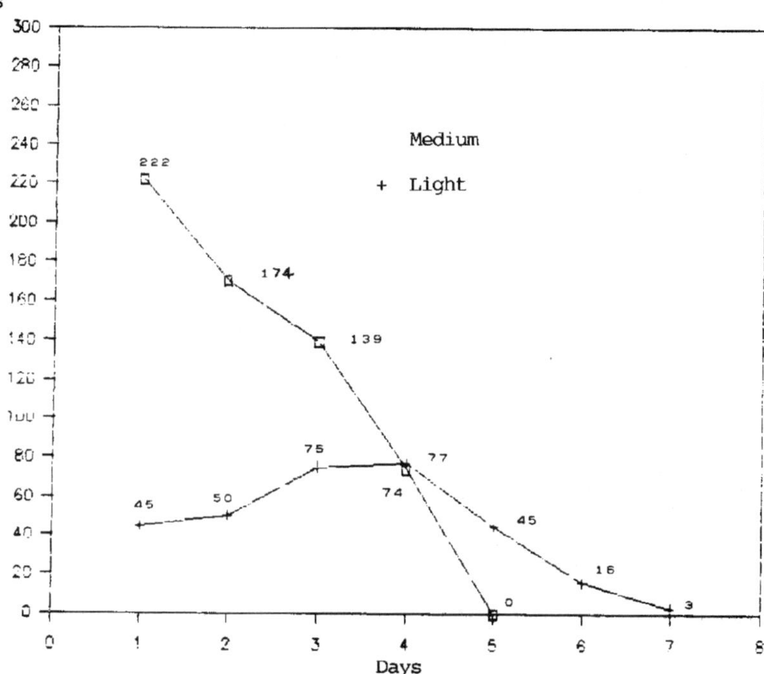

According to the analysis from the "graph of the total subjects'
daily changes of the degrees of severity of symptoms" constructed from
statistical data, XH-1 drug addiction therapy has conspicuous suppressing
effect on heroin quitters' severe withdrawal reaction of the 3rd and 4th day.

THE DAILY STATISTICAL CHART OF   (6-1)
THE TOTAL GROUP POPULATION'S
REHABILITATING DEGREE OF HEALTH ITEMS   No. of participants: 94

Health Items	Degree of Rehabilitation		
	good	fair	poor
food appetite	88	5	1
sleep	82	11	1
spirited feel after awakening	65	28	1
physical strength	68	24	2
degree of comfort symptom .	61	32	1
sexual appetite	8	29	57
Statistics	372	129	63

Whether there is anyone with withdrawal reaction.

THE DAILY STATISTICAL CHART OF   (6-2)
THE TOTAL GROUP POPULATION'S
REHABILITATING DEGREE OF HEALTH ITEMS   No. of participants: 94

Health Items	Degree of Rehabilitation		
	good	fair	poor
food appetite	90	4	0
sleep	85	8	1
spirited feel after awakening	75	18	1
physical strength	76	17	1
degree of comfort symptom	68	25	1
sexual appetite	19	33	42
Statistics	413	105	46

Whether there is anyone with withdrawal reaction.

THE DAILY STATISTICAL CHART OF   (6-3)
THE TOTAL GROUP POPULATION'S
REHABILITATING DEGREE OF HEALTH ITEMS   No. of participants: 94

Health Items	Degree of Rehabilitation		
	good	fair	poor
food appetite	92	2	0
sleep	87	7	0
spirited feel after awakening	84	10	0
physical strength	79	15	0
degree of comfort symptom	73	21	0
sexual appetite	28	35	31
Statistics	443	90	31

Whether there is anyone with withdrawal reaction.

THE DAILY STATISTICAL CHART OF   **(6-4)**
THE TOTAL GROUP POPULATION'S
REHABILITATING DEGREE OF HEALTH ITEMS   No. of participants: 94

Health Items	Degree of Rehabilitation		
	good	fair	poor
food appetite	94	0	0
sleep	91	3	0
spirited feel after awakening	90	4	0
physical strength	83	11	0
degree of comfort symptom ·	81	13	0
sexual appetite	40	43	11
Statistics	479	74	11

Whether there is anyone with withdrawal reaction.

THE DAILY STATISTICAL CHART OF   (6-5)
THE TOTAL GROUP POPULATION'S
REHABILITATING DEGREE OF HEALTH ITEMS   No. of participants: 94

Health Items	Degree of Rehabilitation		
	good	fair	poor
food appetite	94	0	0
sleep	92	2	0
spirited feel after awakening	91	3	0
physical strength	87	7	0
degree of comfort symptom	86	8	0
sexual appetite	64	25	5
Statistics	514	45	5

Whether there is anyone with withdrawal reaction.

THE DAILY STATISTICAL CHART OF   (6-6)
THE TOTAL GROUP POPULATION'S
REHABILITATING DEGREE OF HEALTH ITEMS   No. of participants: 94

Health Items	Degree of Rehabilitation		
	good	fair	poor
food appetite	94	0	0
sleep	92	2	0
spirited feel after awakening	92	2	0
physical strength	89	5	0
degree of comfort symptom	89	5	0
sexual appetite	82	10	2
Statistics	538	24	2

Whether there is anyone with withdrawal reaction.

THE DAILY STATISTICAL CHART OF   (6-7)
THE TOTAL GROUP POPULATION'S
REHABILITATING DEGREE OF HEALTH ITEMS   No. of participants: **94**

Health Items	Degree of Rehabilitation		
	good	fair	poor
food appetite	94	0	0
sleep	92	2	0
spirited feel after awakening	92	2	0
physical strength	90	4	0
degree of comfort symptom	90	4	0
sexual appetite	83	9	2
Statistics	541	21	2

Whether there is anyone with withdrawal reaction.

Each item's group population is   94

      6 items' group population   = 564

Population with good rehabilitating degree = 541

    564 : 541 = 100 : X   = 95.9%

Rate for good rehabilitating effect is 95.9%

    564 : 21 = 100 : X   = 3.7%

Rate for fair rehabilitating effect is 3.7%

        95.9+3.7   = 99.6%

    The total rehabilitating effect is 99.6%

GRAPH OF THE GROUP POPULATION'S DAILY CHANGING TENDENCY
OF THE HEALTH ITEMS IN TERMS OF GOOD, FAIR, AND POOR"

"GRAPH OF THE GROUP POPULATION'S DAILY CHANGING TENDENCY   (7-1)
OF FOOD APPETITE IN TERMS OF GOOD, FAIR, AND POOR"

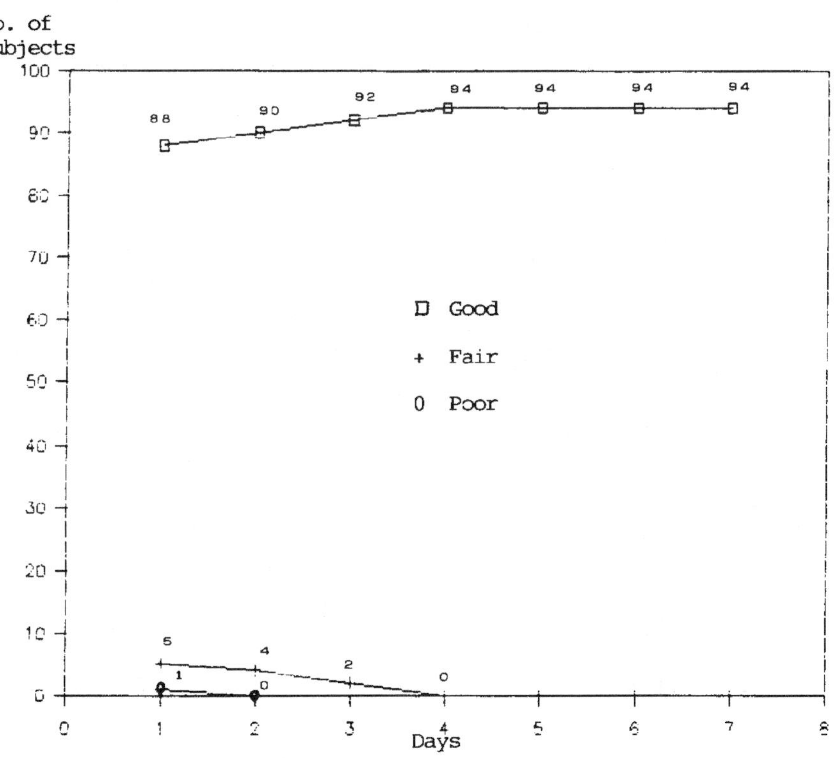

GRAPH OF THE GROUP POPULATION'S DAILY CHANGING TENDENCY
OF THE HEALTH ITEMS IN TERMS OF GOOD, FAIR, AND POOR

"GRAPH OF THE GROUP POPULATION'S DAILY CHANGING TENDENCY   (7-2)
OF SLEEP IN TERMS OF GOOD, FAIR, AND POOR"

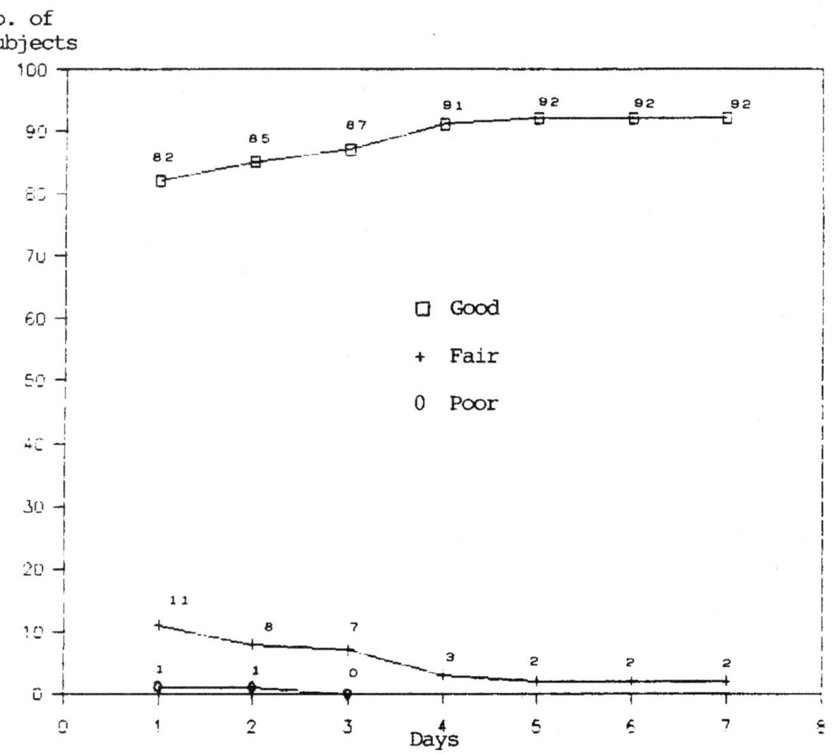

GRAPH OF THE GROUP POPULATION'S DAILY CHANGING TENDENCY
OF THE HEALTH ITEMS IN TERMS OF GOOD, FAIR, AND POOR

"GRAPH OF THE GROUP POPULATION'S DAILY CHANGING TENDENCY   (7-3)
OF SPIRITED FEEL AFTER AWAKENING IN TERMS OF GOOD, FAIR, AND POOR"

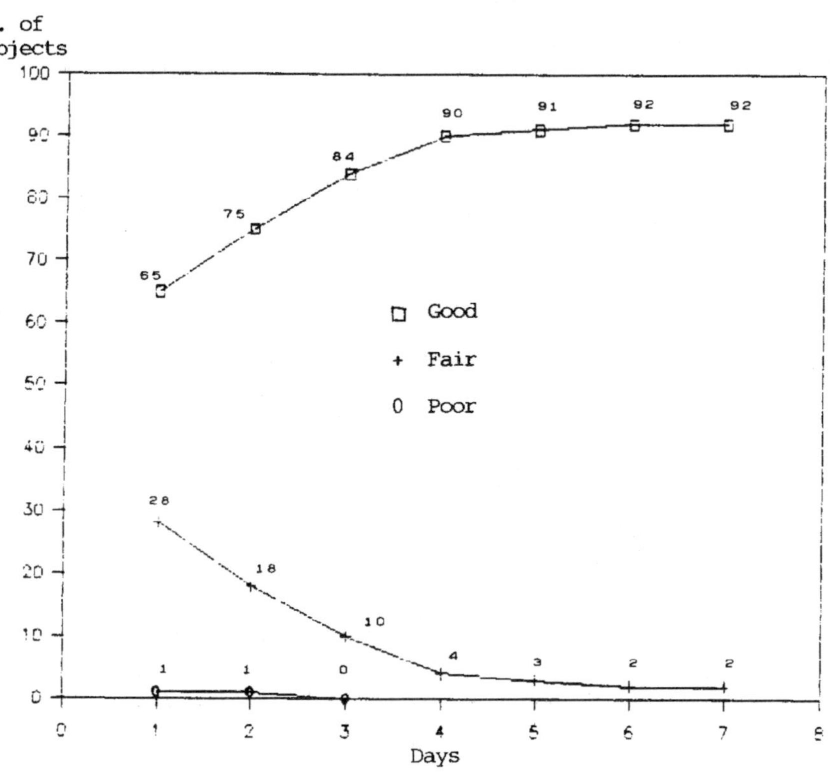

113

GRAPH OF THE GROUP POPULATION'S DAILY CHANGING TENDENCY
OF THE HEALTH ITEMS IN TERMS OF GOOD, FAIR, AND POOR

"GRAPH OF THE GROUP POPULATION'S DAILY CHANGING TENDENCY (7-4)
OF PHYSICAL STRENGTH IN TERMS OF GOOD, FAIR, AND POOR"

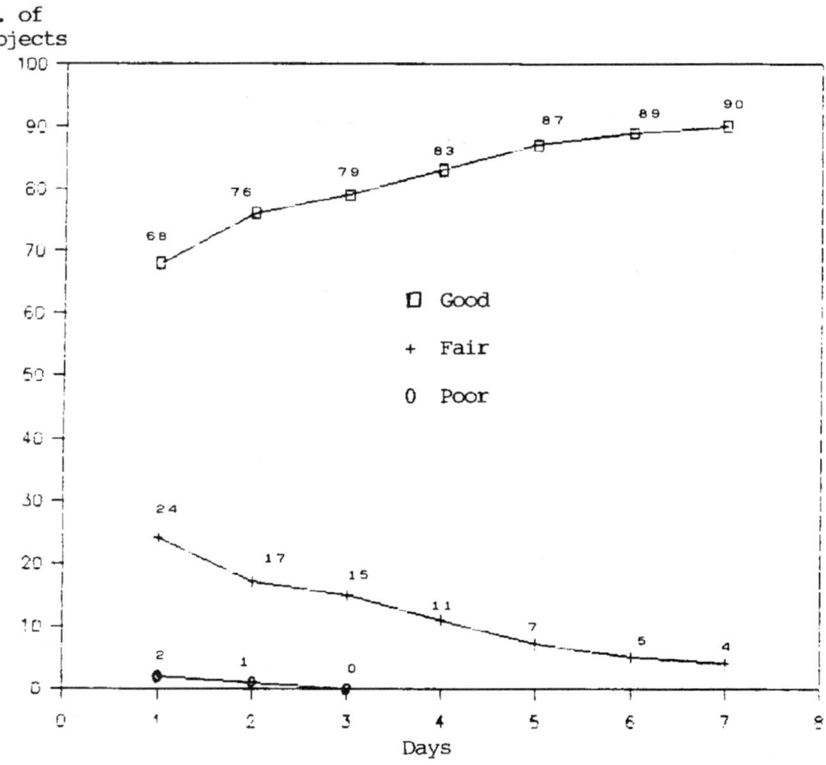

114

GRAPH OF THE GROUP POPULATION'S DAILY CHANGING TENDENCY
OF THE HEALTH ITEMS IN TERMS OF GOOD, FAIR, AND POOR

"GRAPH OF THE GROUP POPULATION'S DAILY CHANGING TENDENCY   (7-5)
OF DEGREE OF COMFORT SYMPTOM IN TERMS OF GOOD, FAIR, AND POOR"

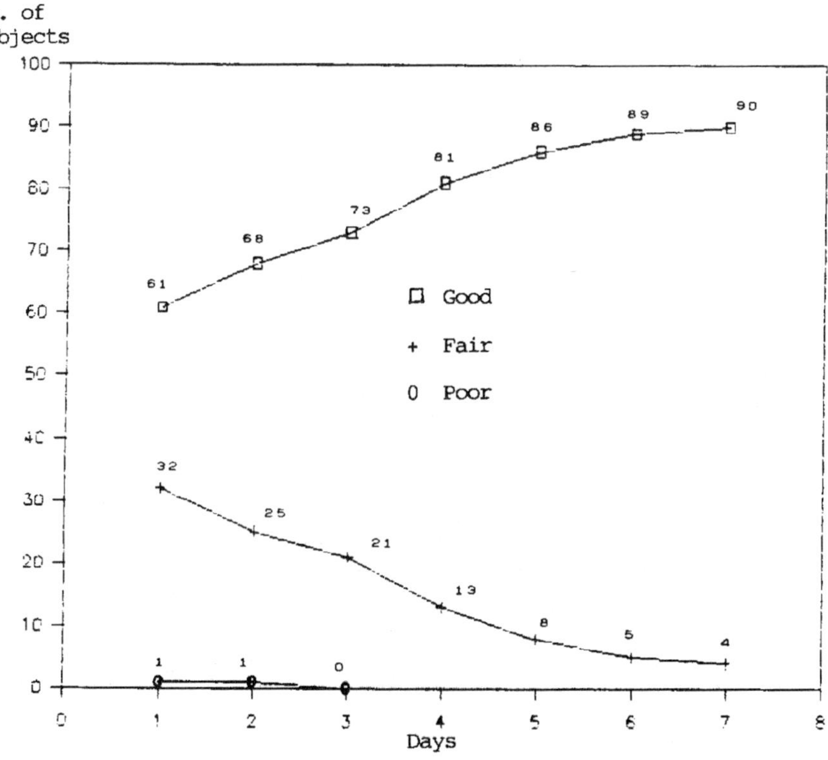

GRAPH OF THE GROUP POPULATION'S DAILY CHANGING TENDENCY
OF THE HEALTH ITEMS IN TERMS OF GOOD, FAIR, AND POOR

"GRAPH OF THE GROUP POPULATION'S DAILY CHANGING TENDENCY   (7-6)
OF SEXUAL APPETITE IN TERMS OF GOOD, FAIR, AND POOR"

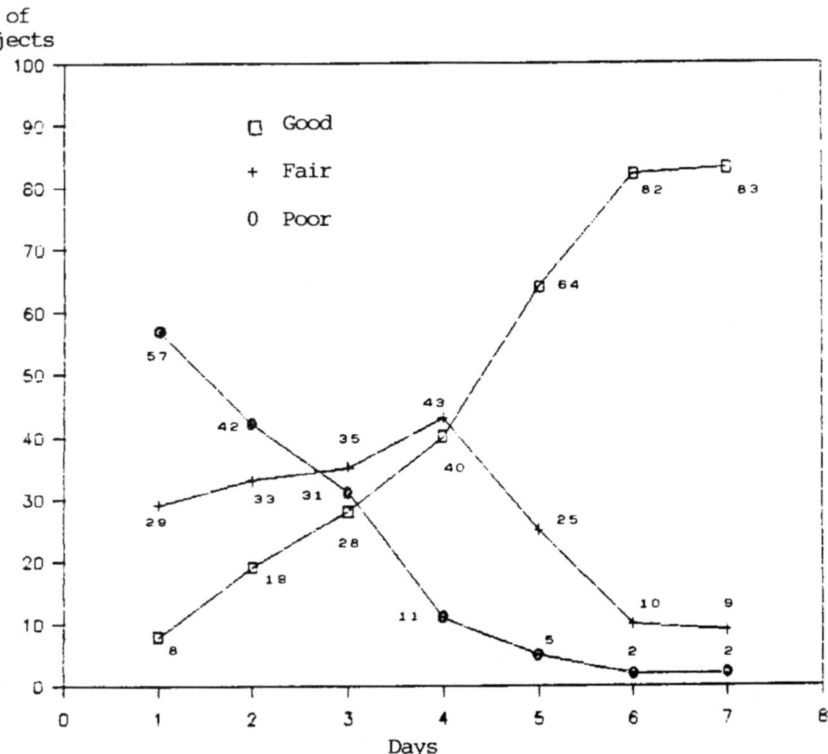

GRAPH OF THE TOTAL GROUP POPULATION'S DAILY CHANGING TENDENCY
OF THE TOTAL HEALTH ITEMS IN TERMS OF GOOD, FAIR, AND POOR

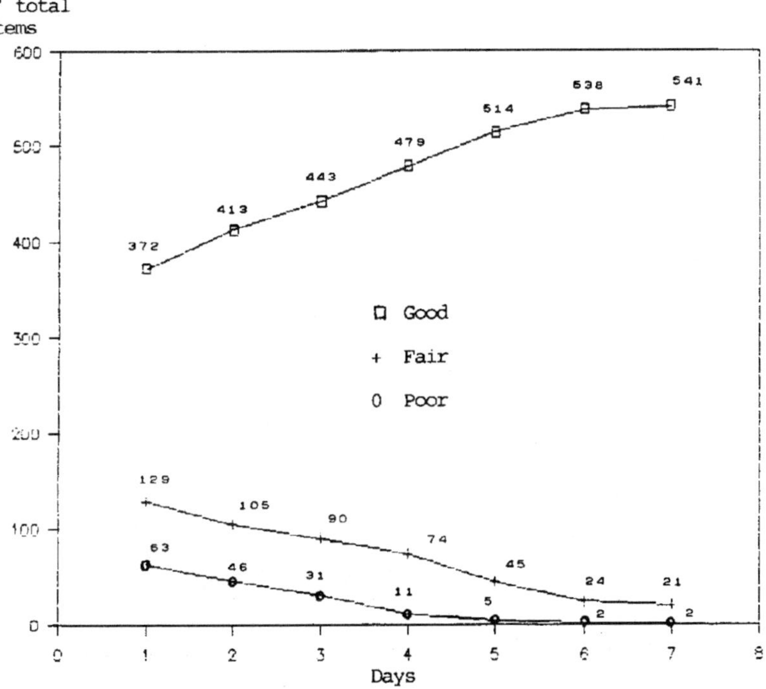

117

GRAPH OF THE DAILY GROUP POPULATION
OF SUBJECTS THAT CRAVE FOR HIGH VOLUME OF FOOD

"THE SPECIAL PHENOMENON DURING THE COURSE OF DRUG ADDICTION TREATMENT"

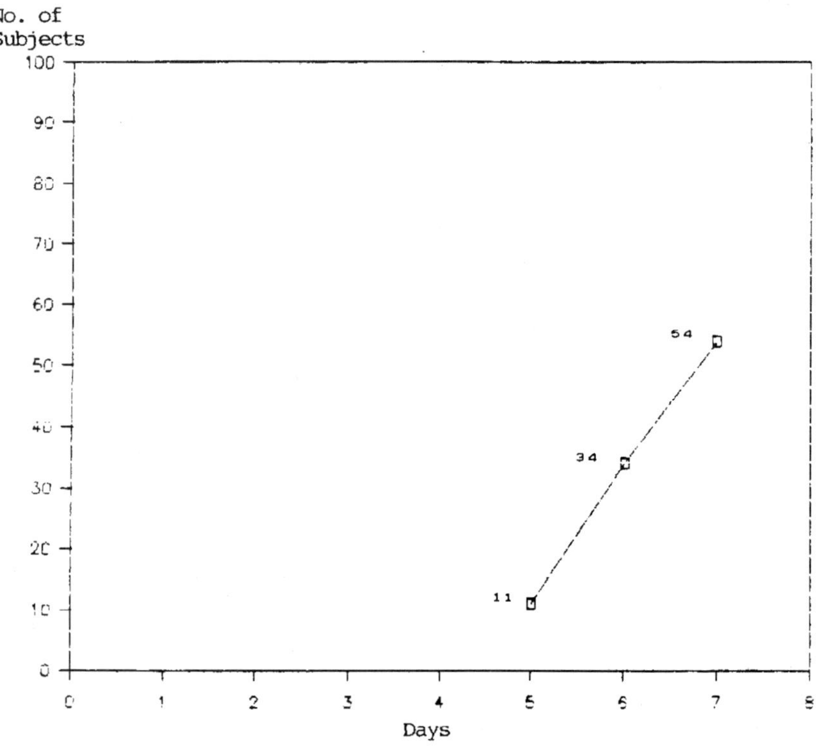

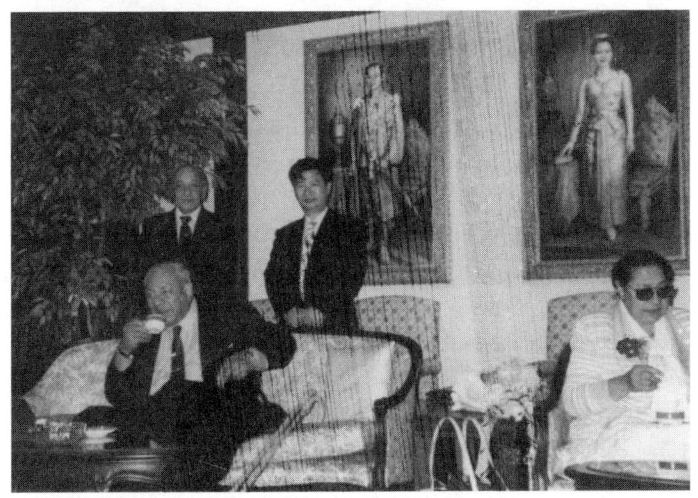

*The King of the Kingdom of Tonga, His Majesty, King Taufa'ahau Tupou IV
(sitting in the front) goes to the Bangkok Metropolitan Administration of
Thailand to especially visit Dr. Laiyin Yan and also accepts health treatment of
the XH-1 therapy, which was invented by Dr. Laiyin Yan. In the picture: The
King of Tonga is resting in Bangkok Airport V.I.P. room. (Sitting on the right)
The Queen of the Kingdom of Tonga, Her Majesty, Halaevalu Matá aho.
(Standing in the right rear) Dr. Laiyin Yan, royal physician of the Kingdom of
Tonga, who is also a specialized physician of the Republic of China, vice-
president and research professor of California Medical Research Institute of
U.S.A., and advisor of the BMA Drug Addicts Treatment Program. (Standing
in the left rear) Dr. Tili Puloka, royal physician of the Kingdom of Tonga, who is
also advisor to the California Medical Research Institute of U.S.A.*

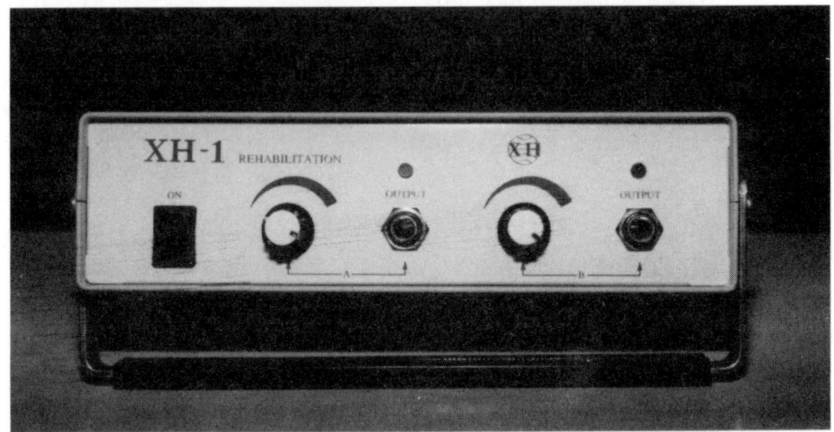

*This is the XH-1 rehabilitation therapeutic machine, which is famous
worldwide in each country's department of health and has an efficacy rate of
at least 90 percent on treating twenty-one types of illnesses.*

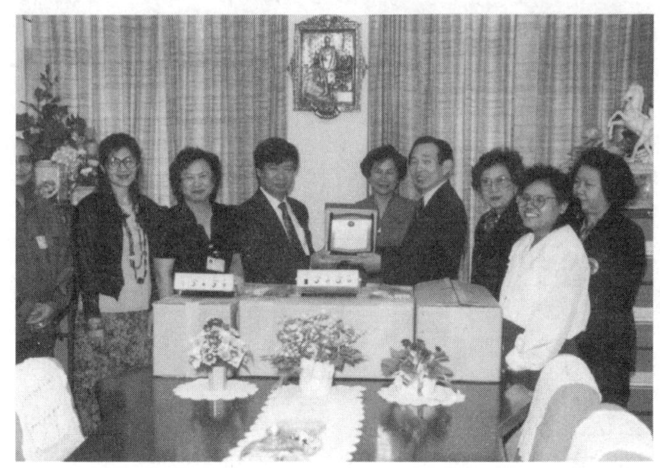

Bangkok Metropolitan Administration compliments Dr. Laiyin Yan (fourth left), for eight years of assisting Bangkok Metropolitan Administration on using XH-1 to treat illnesses and drug addiction and his outstanding accomplishments by awarding him a gold medal. (4th right) Dr. Kachit Choopanya, Deputy Permanent Secretary on Public Health of the Bangkok Metropolitan Administration. (3rd right) Dr. Su Vanichseni, Vice-president of the Department of Health of the Bangkok Metropolitan Administration. (Center) Dr. Swanee Raktham, in charge of Drug Prevention and Treatment Center of the Bangkok Metropolitan Administration. (3rd left) Ms. Suneeporn Anuttarakulvanich, in charge of the 12th Narcotic Clinic of the Bangkok Metropolitan Administration.

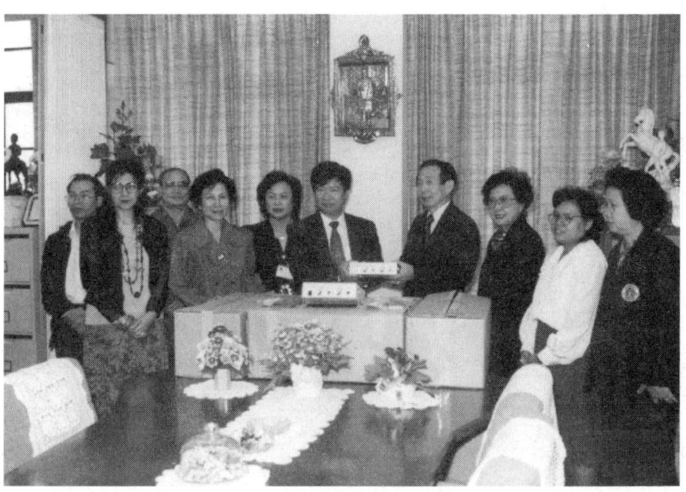

Bangkok Metropolitan Administration receives Twenty XH-1 rehabilitation therapeutic machines given by the Vice-president of California Medical Research Institute of U.S.A., Dr. Laiyin Yan.

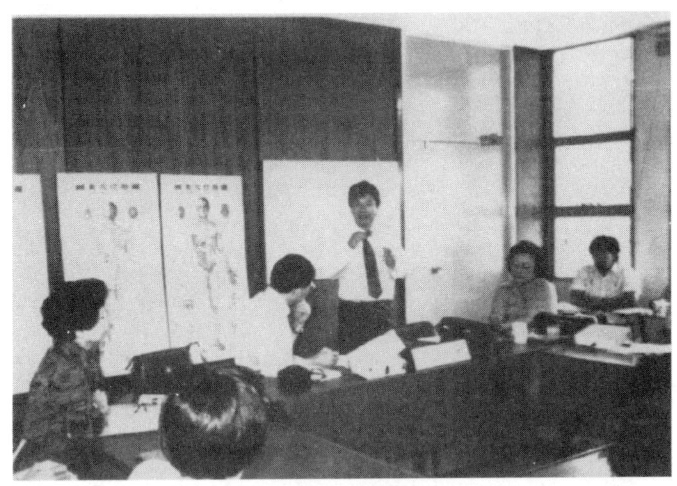

Dr. Laiyin Yan is training medical staffs of Bangkok Metropolitan Administration in how to use XH-1 illness and drug-addiction therapy. (First left) Person in charge of the Drug Prevention and Treatment Center of Bangkok Metropolitan Administration, Dr. Suwanee Raktham. (Second right) Person in charge of the Twelfth Narcotic Clinic of Bangkok Metropolitan Administration, Ms. Suneeporn Anuttarakulvanich.

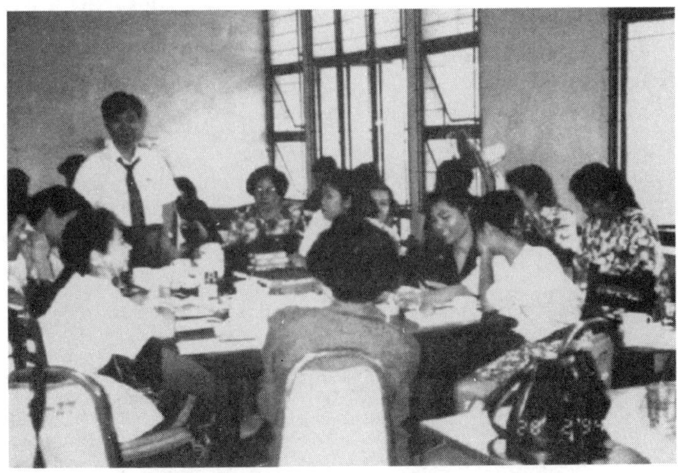

Medical staffs of Bangkok Metropolitan Administration who accept XH-1 illness and drug-addiction therapy are listening to Dr. Laiyin Yan (person standing) lecture and using XH-1 rehabilitation therapeutic machine to treat their own eyes and ears. (1st left) A student is treating her own eyes. (2nd left) A student is treating her own ear.

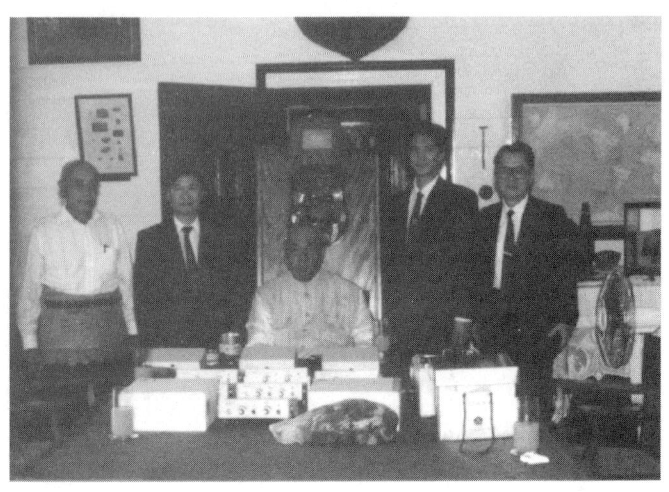

The King of Kingdom of Tonga, His Majesty, King Taufa'ahau Tupou IV (person sitting down) receives Twelve XH-1 rehabilitation therapeutic machines, which are given by the Vice-president of California Medical Research Institute of U.S.A., Dr. Laiyin Yan (second left) and will be distributed to the ministries of health of three countries: Kingdom of Tonga, Nauru, and Tuvalu. (1st right) Mr. Hugh O'Young, Ambassador of the Republic of China at Tonga. (1st left) Dr. Tili Puloka, royal physician of the Kingdom of Tonga, who is also advisor to the California Medical Research Institute of U.S.A. (2nd right) Peter Shieh, Director of California Medical Research Institute of U.S.A.

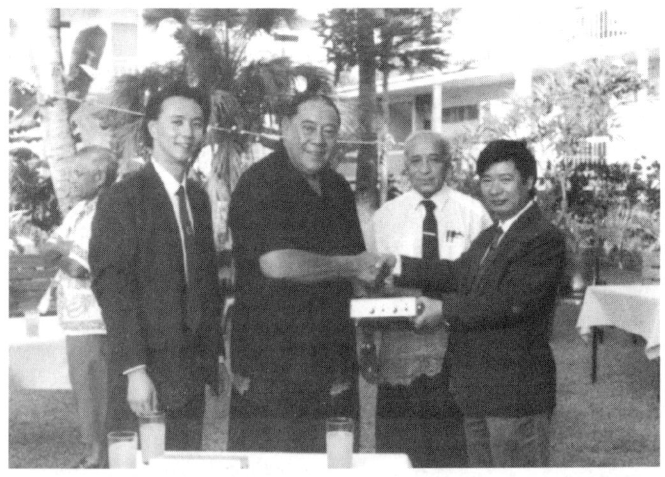

Prime Minister of Kingdom of Tonga, Mr. Baron Vaea (second left), receives XH-1 rehabilitation therapeutic machines given by the Vice-president of California Medical Research Institute of U.S.A., Dr. Laiyin Yan (first right).

At the eighty-people-large welcome cocktail party for Dr. Laiyin Yan (left) given by the Ministry of Health of the Kingdom of Tonga, the Prime Minister of the Kingdom of Tonga, Mr. Baron Vaea (right), is using the green-line electrodes of an XH-1 rehabilitation therapeutic machine to treat his own eyes.

At the eighty-people-large welcome cocktail party for Dr. Laiyin Yan (left) given by the Ministry of Health of Kingdom of the Tonga, the Ambassador of the Republic of China at Tonga, Mr. Hugh O'Young (second right), is using the green-line electrodes of an XH-1 rehabilitation therapeutic machine to treat his own eyes. (First left) Director of California Medical Research Institute of U.S.A., Peter Shieh.

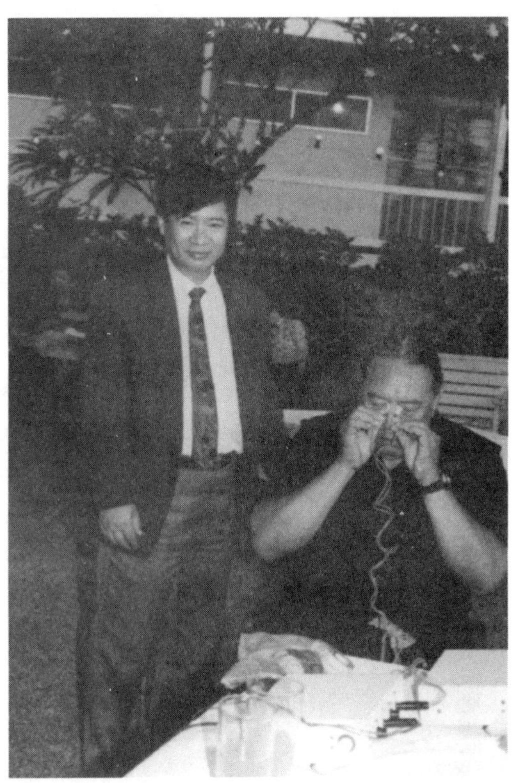

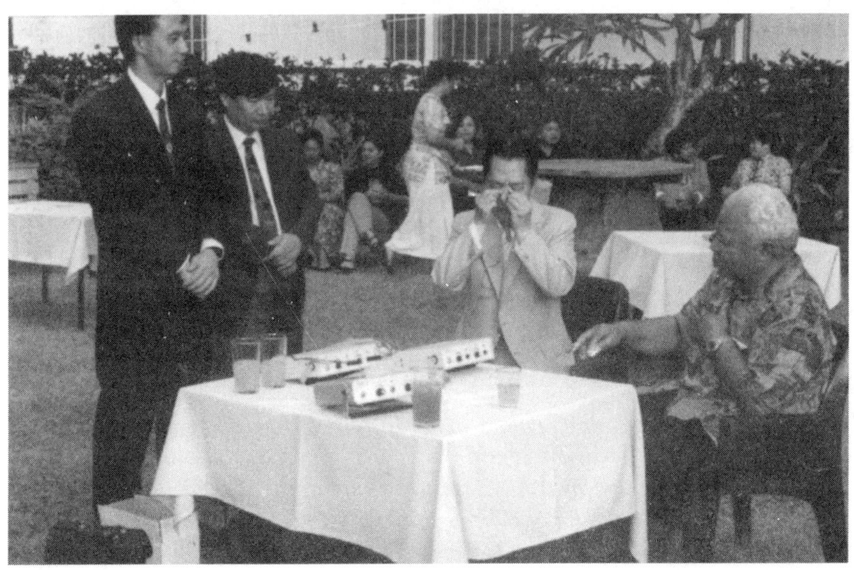

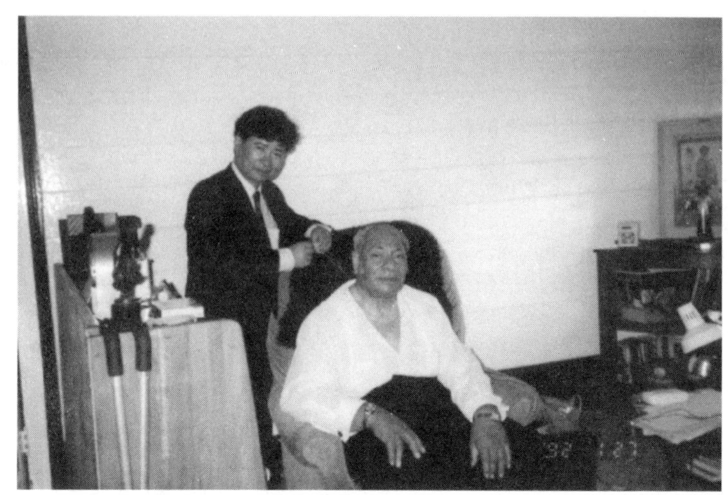

In the Kingdom of Tonga, Dr. Laiyin Yan used XH-1 therapy and cured His Majesty King Taufa'ahau Tupou IV's cervical disorder and pains in the leg joints.

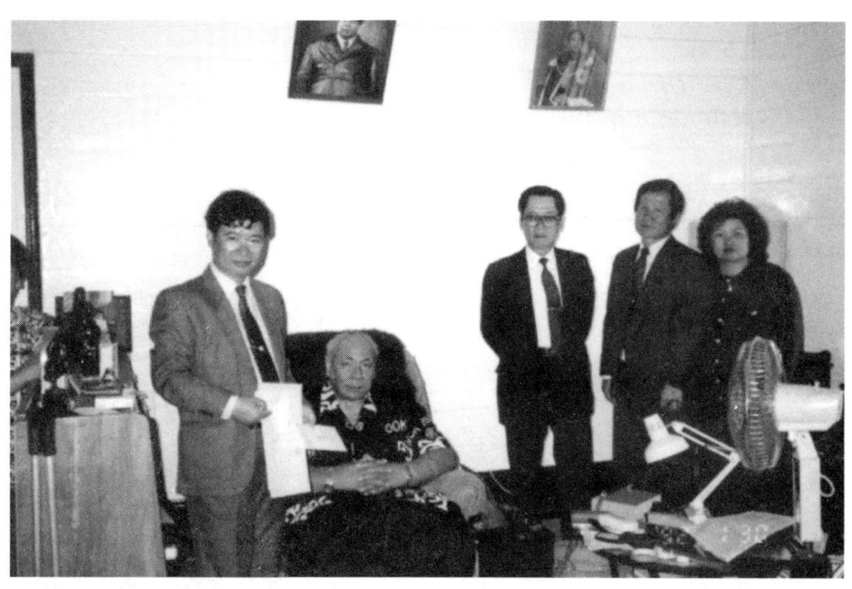

The King of the Kingdom of Tonga, His Majesty, King Taufa'ahau Tupou IV (sitting in the rear), issued a certificate which gives Dr. Laiyin Yan (first left) the official title as Royal Physician of Kingdom of Tonga. (Third right) Ambassador of the Republic of China at Tonga, Mr. Hugh O'Young.

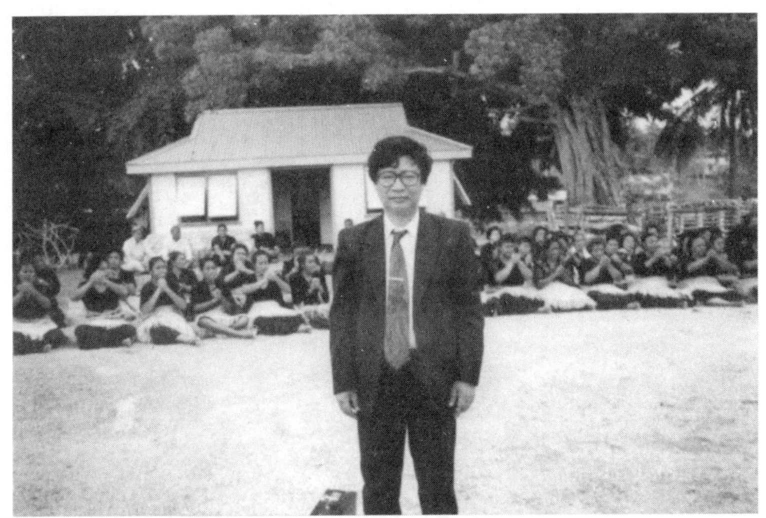

On September 16, 1991, Kingdom of Tonga, HRH Prince 'Aho'eitu was appointed Noble 'Ulukalala. At the ceremony of inauguration, Dr. Laiyin Yan, due to having cured the King of Tonga, His Majesty, King Taufa'ahau Tupou IV's illness in two days by using the self-invented XH-1 therapy, was chosen as the most knowledgeable and respectable foreigner of the Kingdom of Tonga over the last thirty-two years and to present the gift to the King of Tonga. In the picture: Dr. Laiyin Yan is given a welcome at the Palace.

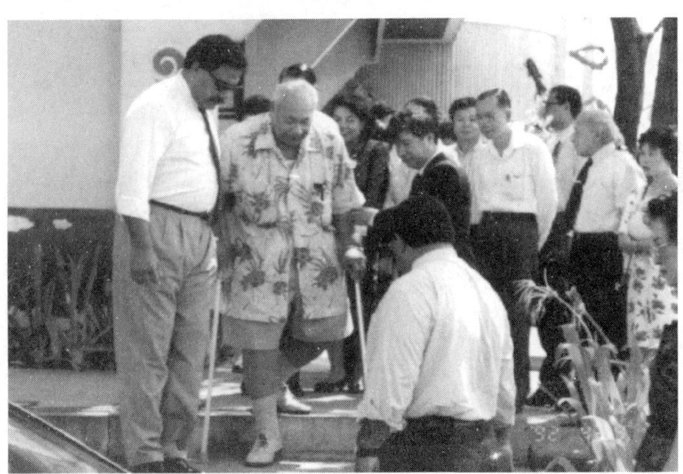

The King of the Kingdom of Tonga, His Majesty, King Taufa'ahau Tupou IV went to the Nineteenth Medical Clinic of Bangkok Metropolitan Administration to especially visit Dr. Laiyin Yan and accepted three XH-1 rehabilitation therapeutic machines given by Bangkok Metropolitan Administration. In the picture: Dr. Laiyin Yan is holding the King of Tonga while walking.

125

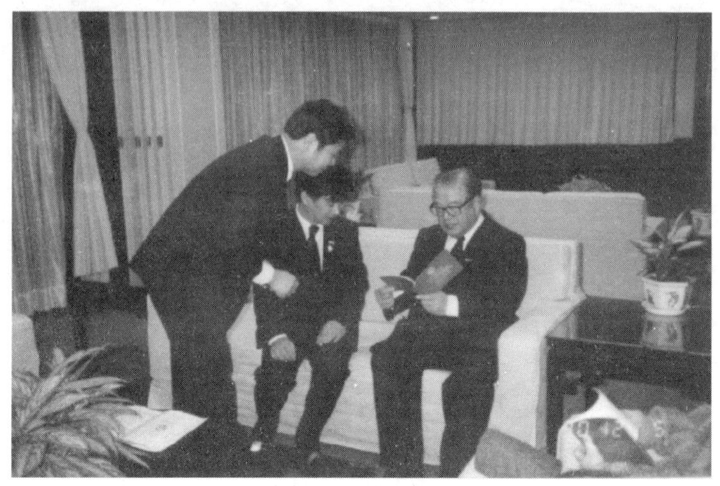

At the airport V.I.P. room, Secretary-General to the president of the Republic of China, Mr. Yien-shi Tsiang (sitting to the right), receives specialized physician of the Republic of China, Dr. Laiyin Yan (sitting in the center), for more than an hour and gives attention to the Dr. Laiyin Yan-invented medication-free XH-1 illness and drug-addiction therapy.

Director-General of the Department of Health of the Republic of China, Dr. Po-ya Chang (left) receives representative staff of Bangkok Metropolitan Administration, who is also advisor of BMA Drug Addicts Treatment Program, Dr. Laiyin Yan (right), and gives attention to the medication-free XH-1 illness and drug-addiction therapy.

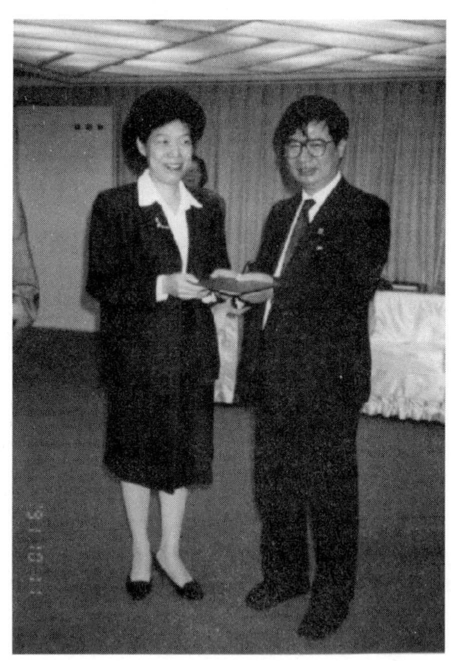

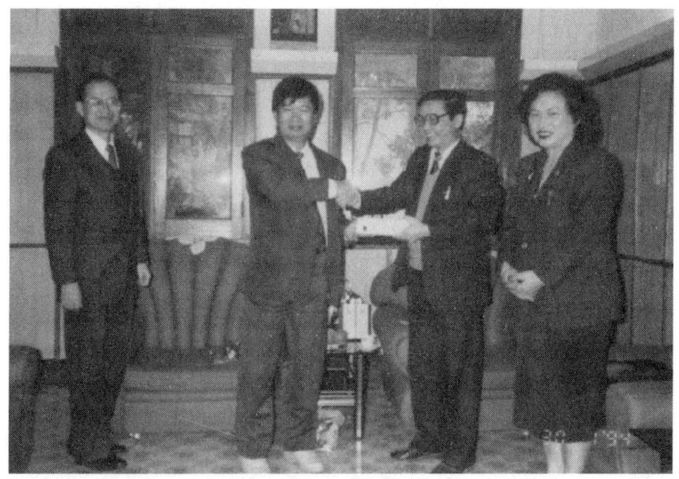

Vice-minister of Vietnam's Ministry of Public Health, Le Ngoc Trong (second right), accepts five XH-1 rehabilitation therapeutic machines given by specialized physician of the Republic of China, who is also vice-president and Research Professor of California Medical Research Institute of U.S.A., Dr. Laiyin Yan (second left). (First left) Representative of the Republic of China's Representative Office at Vietnam, Mr. Sui-chi Lin. (First right) Person in charge of the Twelfth Narcotic Clinic of Bangkok Metropolitan Administration, Ms. Suneeporn Anuttarakulvanich.

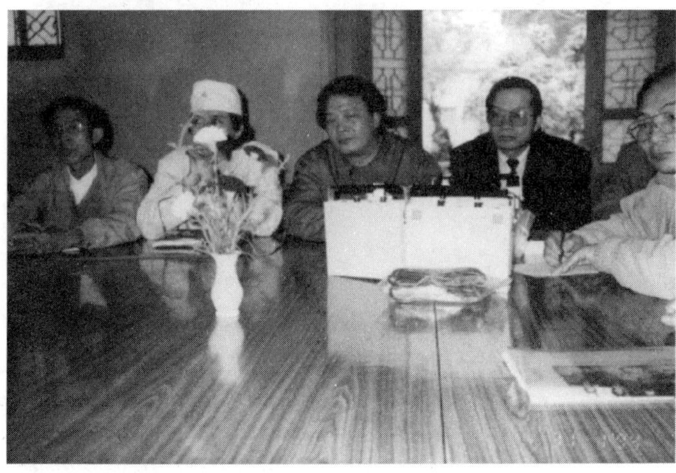

In Vietnam, specialized neurologists of Ministry of Public Health are listening to Dr. Laiyin Yan lecturing on XH-1 illness and drug-addiction therapy.

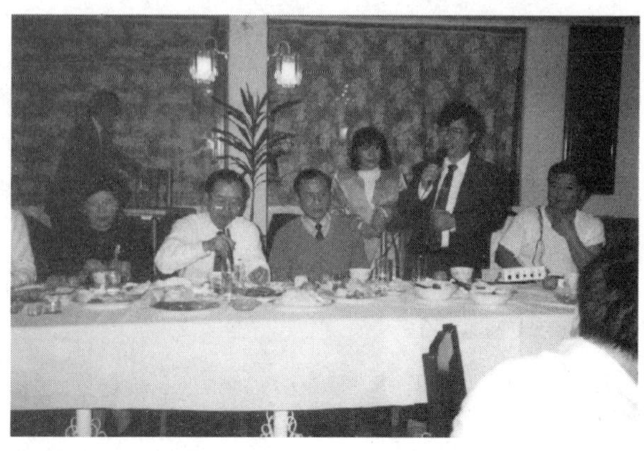

At the seventy-six-people-large welcome feast celebrated by the Representative of the Republic of China's Representative Office at Vietnam, Mr. Sui-chi Lin (second left) for specialized physician of the Republic of China, who is also vice-president and research professor of California Medical Research Institute of U.S.A., Dr. Laiyin Yan (second right). Dr. Laiyin Yan is introducing the XH-1 illness and drug-addiction therapy to Vietnam's well-known people from each field. (Center) Head of the International Cooperative Bureau of Vietnam's Ministry of Public Health. (1st left) Representative Mr. Sui-chi Lin's first lady. (1st right) President of Vietnam's Taiwan Guildhall.

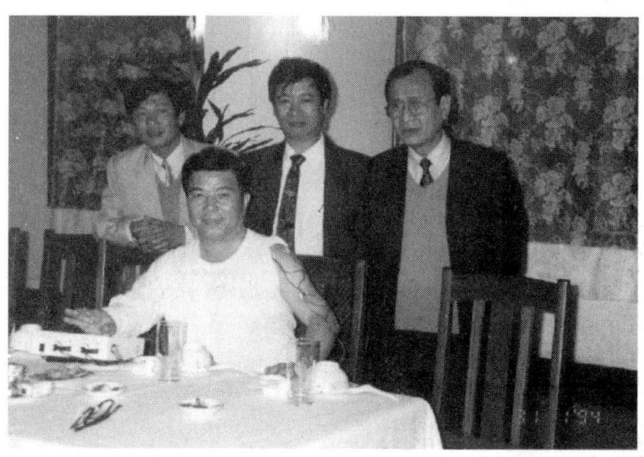

President of Taiwan Guildhall (person sitting down) had shoulder periarthritis for more than half a year, could not raise either arm, and could not put on clothes by himself. At the feast, he asked Dr. Laiyin Yan (center rear) to use the XH-1 rehabilitation therapeutic machine to treat him. In one hour, both of his arms could be raised and he was no longer in pain. (1st right rear) Head of the International Cooperative Bureau of Vietnam's Ministry of Public Health. (1st left rear) Specialized neurologist of Vietnam.

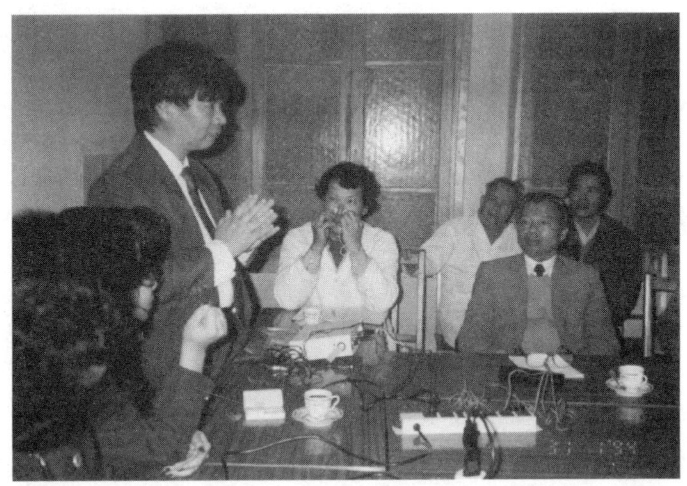

Dr. Laiyin Yan (person standing) lecturing in Vietnam to the specialized neurologists of the Ministry of Public Health on XH-1 illness and drug-addiction therapy. A physician under training (center) is using an XH-1 rehabilitation therapeutic machine to treat his own rhinitis and achieved a very good effect in fifteen minutes.

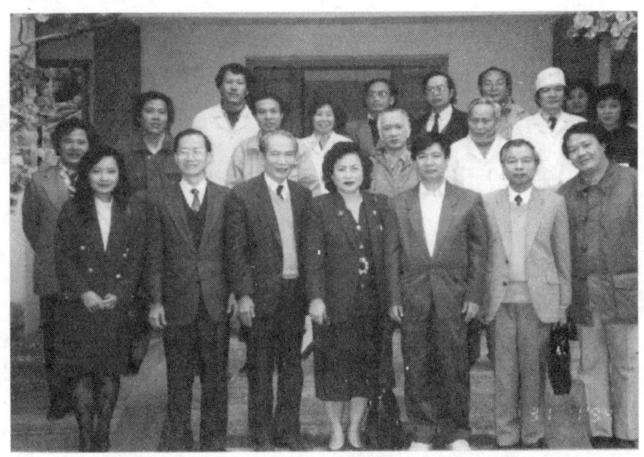

Dr. Laiyin Yan (third right), pictured together with all of Vietnam's Ministry of Public Health physicians who received the XH-1 illness and drug-addiction therapy training. (Third left) President of Vietnam's National Association of Psychiatry, Neurology, and Neurosurgery, Pr. Nguyen Viet. (Second left) Representative of the Republic of China's Representative Office at Vietnam, Mr. Sui-chi Lin. (Center) Person in charge of the Twelfth Narcotic Clinic of Bangkok Metropolitan Administration, Ms. Suneeporn Anuttarakulvanich.

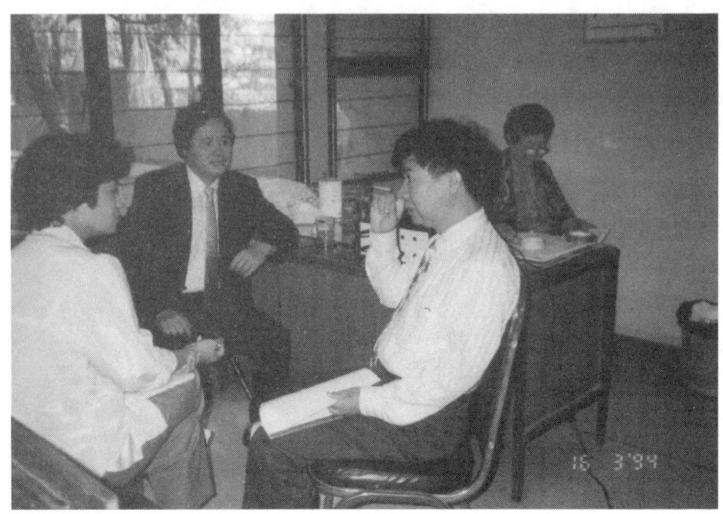

Specialized neurologists sent from Vietnam's Ministry of Health to Bangkok Metropolitan Administration to learn XH-1 illness and drug-addiction therapy are accepting advisor of BMA Drug Addicts Treatment Program, Dr. Laiyin Yan's (right) training. (Center) Dr. Ngo Thanh Hoi. (Left) Dr. Luu To Phan.

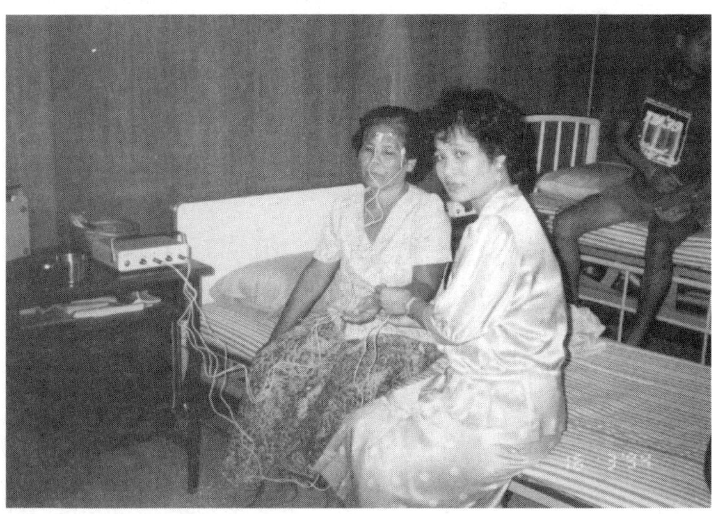

Specialized neurologist, Dr. Luu To Phan, sent from Vietnam's Ministry of Public Health to Bangkok Metropolitan Administration to learn XH-1 illness and drug-addiction therapy, is using the yellow-line electrodes of the XH-1 rehabilitation therapeutic machine to treat migraine on a patient.

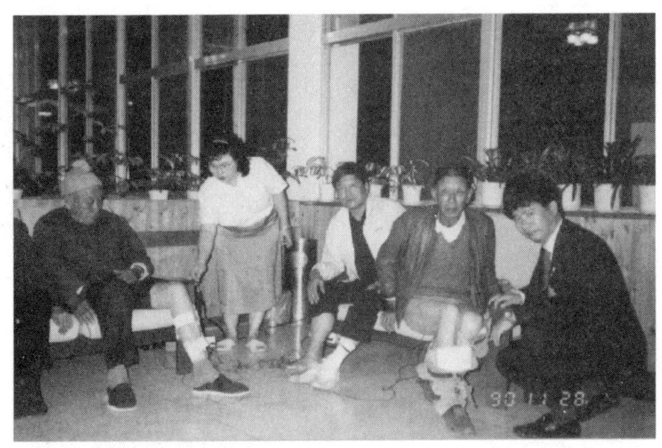

At the third Joint Conference of the World Congress of Chinese Medicine and Acupuncture gathered together in Taipei, person in charge of the Twelfth Narcotic Clinic of Bangkok Metropolitan Administration, Ms. Suneeporn Anuttarakulvanich (second left), is using XH-1 rehabilitation therapeutic machine to treat a patient (first left), whose left leg has been paralyzed for three years. Dr. Laiyin Yan (first right), is diagnosing the condition of the patient's illness.

The patient, whose left leg has been paralyzed for three years, after thirty minutes of treatment using XH-1 rehabilitation therapeutic machine, can stand up and walk.

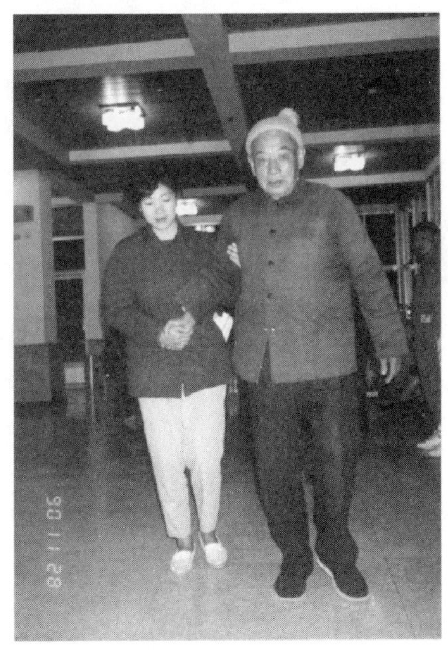

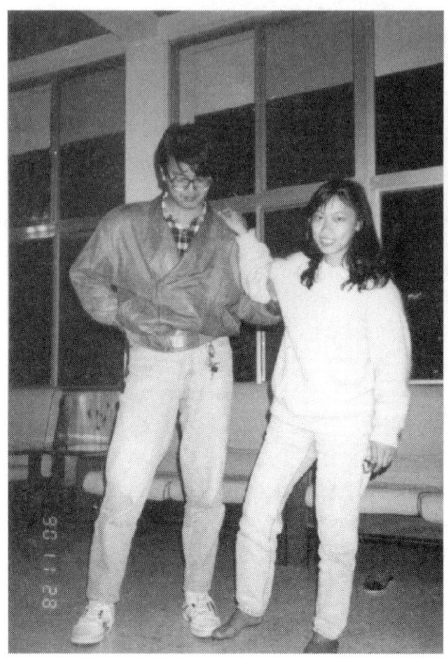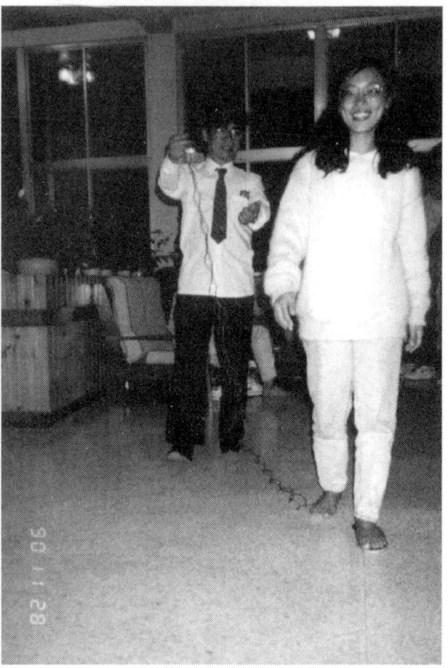

In the left picture: At the third Joint Conference of the World Congress of Chinese Medicine and Acupuncture gather together in Taipei, a female student has a sprained ankle and is unable to walk. In order to walk, she needs to be held by someone else.

In the right picture: After being treated for thirty minutes by Dr. Laiyin Yan (rear), using the self-invented XH-1 rehabilitation therapeutic machine, she can start walking.

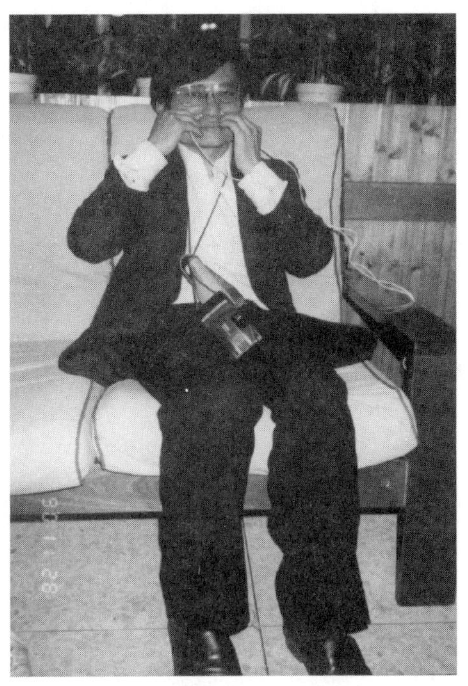

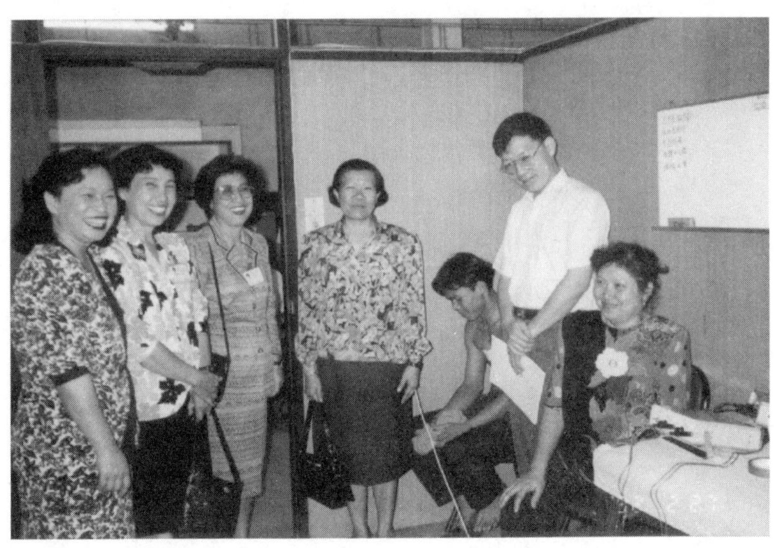

Vice-president of Department of Health of Bangkok Metropolitan Administration, Dr. Su Vanichsenee (third left), is observing the condition of using XH-1 illness and drug-addiction therapy to treat illnesses.

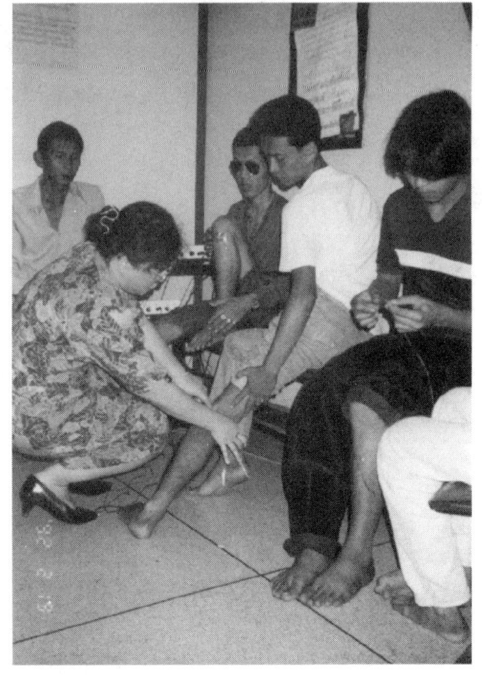

Person in charge of the Twelfth Narcotic Clinic of Bangkok Metropolitan Administration, Ms. Suneeporn Anuttarakulvanich (second left), is using XH-1 illness and drug-addiction therapy to treat a drug quitter's leg cramp. A drug quitter (first right) is using the blue-line electrodes of XH-1 rehabilitation therapeutic machine to treat drug addiction on himself.

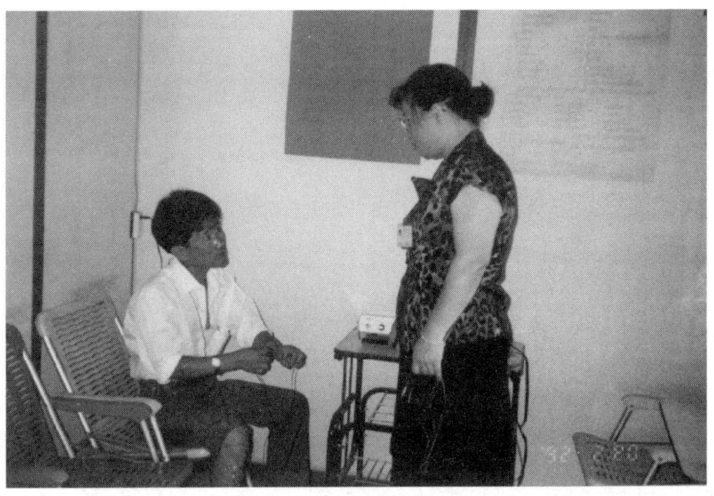

Person in charge of the Twelfth Narcotic Clinic of Bangkok Metropolitan Administration, Ms. Suneeporn Anuttarakulvanich, (person standing), is training a drug quitter (person sitting) on how to use the blue-line electrodes of the XH-1 rehabilitation therapeutic machine to treat drug addiction on himself.

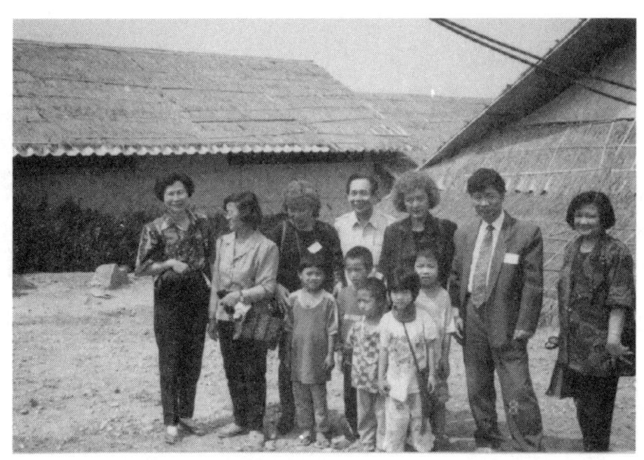

Advisor of BMA Drug Addicts Treatment Program, Dr. Laiyin Yan (second right), senior officials of Bangkok Metropolitan Administration, and the main drug-addiction treating staffs go to the Golden Triangle to investigate drugs (Center) Deputy Permanent Secretary on Public Health of Bangkok Metropolitan Administration, Dr. Kachit Choopanya (First left) Person in charge of the Drug Prevention and Treatment Center of Bangkok Metropolitan Administration, Dr. Suwanee Raktham. (Third left) Person in charge of the Twelfth Narcotic Clinic of Bangkok Metropolitan Administration, Ms. Suneeporn Anuttarakulvanich.

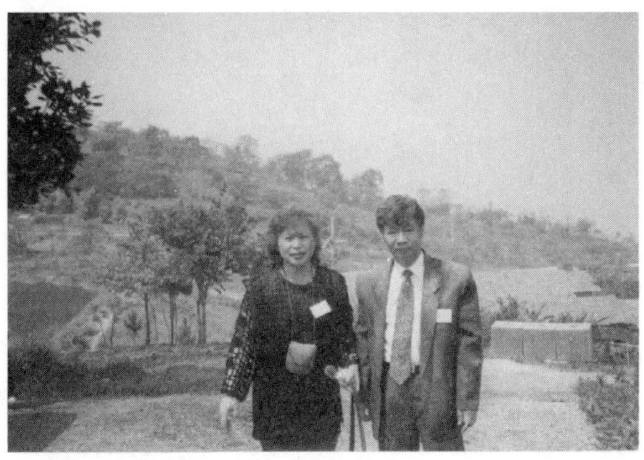

Advisor of BMA Drug Addicts Treatment Program, Dr. Laiyin Yan, and person in charge of the Twelfth Narcotic Clinic of Bangkok Metropolitan Administration Ms. Suneeporn Anuttarakulvanich, are in the Golden Triangle to investigate drugs.

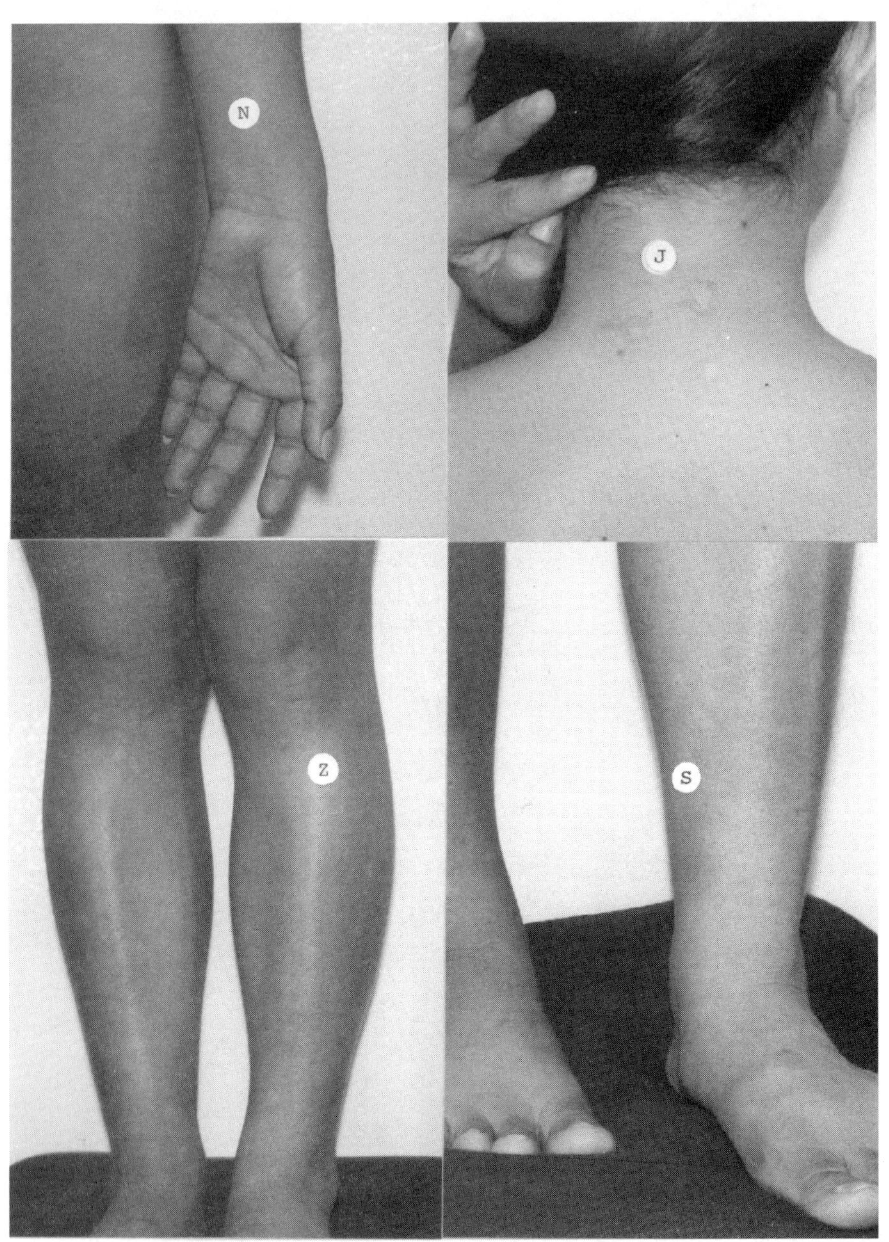

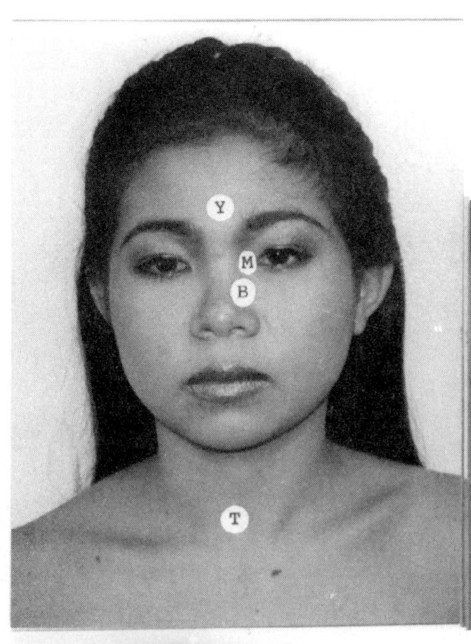

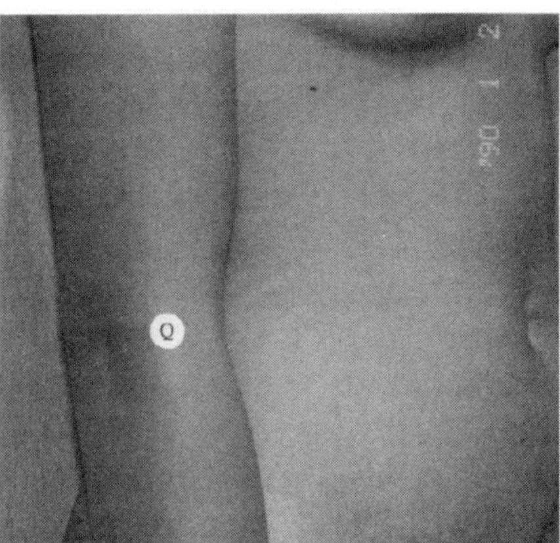

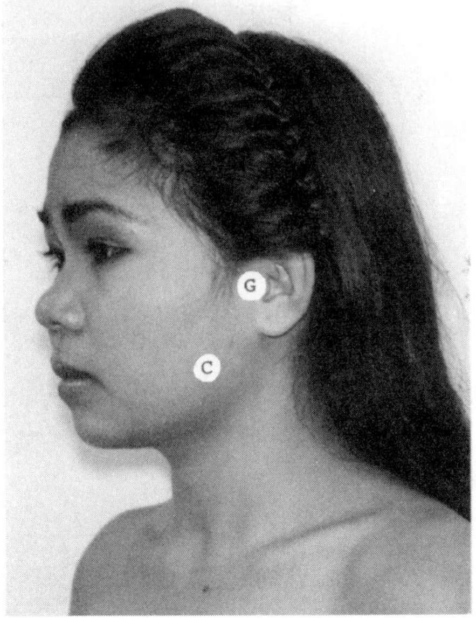